The Which? Guide to
Men's Health

About the Author

Dr Steve Carroll MB, BS, MRCS, LRCP is a former GP who now writes full-time on medical and health issues for both professional and consumer audiences. In addition to the many articles he has had published in magazines such as *Bella* and *Which? way to Health*, Dr Carroll is the author of *The Complete Family Guide to Healthy Living* and has contributed to several other health books. Before turning his hand to writing, Dr Carroll worked in sports medicine: he was previously Assistant Team Doctor to Tottenham Hotspur Football Club and Expedition Doctor for the Ian Botham Hannibal Charity Trek across the Alps. He is currently a director of CPR Worldwide Ltd, a leading international healthcare communications consultancy.

The Which? Guide to Men's Health

Dr Steve Carroll

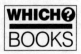 CONSUMERS' ASSOCIATION

Which? Books are commissioned by
Consumers' Association and published by
Which? Ltd, 2 Marylebone Road,
London NW1 4DF
Email address: books@which.net

Distributed by The Penguin Group:
Penguin Books Ltd, 27 Wrights Lane, London W8 5TZ

First edition June 1994
Revised edition September 1995
Reprinted 1997
Revised edition January 1999

British Library Cataloguing-in-Publication Data
A catalogue record for this book is available from the British Library

ISBN 0 85202 758 3

For a full list of Which? books, please write to Which? Books, Castlemead,
Gascoyne Way, Hertford X, SG14 1LH, or access our web site at
www.which.net

Cover and text design by Kyzen Creative Consultants
Text illustrations by Andrew Bezear

Typeset by Business ColorPrint Ltd, Welshpool, Powys, Wales
Printed in Great Britain by Clays Ltd, Bungay, Suffolk

Contents

Introduction

We never anticipate that bad health is something waiting to happen to us, although we know it happens to other people. But illness or disease can strike at any time, and, just like a lottery win, it's worth remembering that 'It could be you'. Recently, I discovered that to my cost.

I trained for 10 years to become a GP. I then spent another 10 years writing books and magazine articles designed to try to make people more aware of their own health. But being a typical male myself, I chose to ignore my own advice and do nothing about the tiny lump that had appeared on the right side of my nose in 1996.

I suppose I just became used to my lump. I saw it every day in the mirror and, for more than two years, it never caused me any problems. It was smooth, the same colour as the rest of my nose, and once it had reached the size of half a pea, it just stopped growing.

The only reason I finally asked my GP to refer me to a dermatologist was vanity. I was getting married and thought I would rather not see my lump in the wedding photos, even though I had become used to it and I knew my girlfriend loved me – 'lump and all'.

Imagine my horror, and then my guilt, on discovering that, by disobeying one simple piece of health advice – to have any slowly growing skin lump checked out by a doctor – I was now the proud owner of a basal cell carcinoma (rodent ulcer) that I had left untreated for over two years.

The good news was that this is a type of cancer that does not spread to other parts of the body. The bad news was that, by waiting this long to get treatment, the cancer had spread sideways and down on to the cartilage in my nose. According to the specialist, in another few months, the tumour could have started to disfigure my face like a burn.

Like most men, I had subconsciously talked myself into believing that if I ignored a health problem, it, in turn, would not be able to hurt me. The reality was that, had it been treated early, the lump could have been removed easily with virtually no scar.

As I write this introduction to the new edition of *The Which? Guide to Men's Health* I am waiting to have 20 tiny stitches removed from my nose. Even though the surgeon has done an excellent job, I will now have a permanent scar, and it could have been a lot worse.

So what do we men really need to do to improve our chances of staying physically, emotionally and sexually healthy into the new millennium? Clearly we need to change our attitude and stop ignoring the warning symptoms of a health problem. We also need easy access to the kind of health information that will lead us to a more healthy lifestyle, with simple, practical tips on how to take better care of our body, mind and sex life.

Are men still the weaker sex?

Five years have now passed since I sat down to write what became the first edition of *The Which? Guide to Men's Health*. So what of significance has changed during that time to improve the health of men in the UK?

Are men still the weaker sex in terms of dying younger from conditions such as heart disease, stroke and cancer? Women are often wrongly considered to be the weaker sex, but in the UK men are twice as likely to die before they reach the age of 65 (usually from preventable conditions such as heart disease, stroke and certain types of cancer).

In fact, according to the most recent figures available (1995), new-born males in the UK can expect to live to the age of 74 years, while females can expect to live beyond 79 years. Just imagine what you could do with five more years of healthy life.

Women's health may be protected by the female sex hormone oestrogen, but even after the menopause – when levels of this hormone plummet – women still have lower death rates from all the major killer diseases and are four times more likely to live beyond the age of 85.

And what of men's emotional health? Are men still more likely to commit suicide than women? It seems so: of the 3,000 or so suicides officially recorded in England and Wales in 1997, over three times as many involved men, a large number of whom were young, which suggests that men are still tending to neglect their emotional well-being as well as their physical health.

Men behaving badly

Are men behaving more responsibly in terms of protecting themselves against HIV and other sexually transmitted diseases? Despite all the publicity about HIV and AIDS, the safer sex message does not seem to be influencing sexual behaviour significantly. The incidence of gonorrhoea (a reliable yardstick of safer sexual practices), which declined during the 1980s, is once again on the increase. There was a 17 per cent increase in the numbers of men with gonorrhoea attending STD clinics in England and Wales between 1995 and 1996.

Are men still as reluctant to visit their GP? Are men still making a lot of fuss over minor illnesses like a simple cold and then, paradoxically, ignoring a more worrying, persistent symptom like chest pain or indigestion, which could be a warning of a serious disease for which prompt treatment could make a huge difference? Well, according to a survey (published in 1997) conducted by the Royal College of General Practitioners, more than 90 per cent of men consult their GP in a 41-month period. However, a Gallup survey carried out in 1997, in which 839 men were interviewed over the telephone, revealed that:

- 31 per cent would delay seeing their GP until a health problem became more irritating
- 20 per cent would avoid seeing their GP about erectile dysfunction (impotence), 10 per cent if they had an alcohol problem, 8 per cent if they had difficulty passing urine, and 7 per cent if they had a sleeping disorder
- interestingly, 73 per cent would like access to a men's health clinic, and 66 per cent would like to be able to telephone a confidential men's health advice line.

As part of its annual UK National Men's Health Awareness Week, the magazine *Men's Health* carried out a readership survey in April 1998 which showed that:

- 36 per cent of men often feel depressed: work was the main reason for the depression (54 per cent), followed by money worries (47 per cent)

- 24 per cent of the men who often felt depressed said they would do nothing, rather than talk to their partner, friends or family, and 15 per cent said they would just go to the pub.

Why being a man could seriously damage your health

One major difference between the sexes is that men tend, in general, to have much less healthy lifestyles than women. Men are more likely to smoke (although just recently the number of young women who smoke is increasing faster than in any other group). Men are also more likely to drink too much alcohol, take too little exercise, eat a poor diet and fail to cope effectively with stress; all of these factors are known to contribute to the development of a variety of serious illnesses.

In addition, although men may be becoming more aware of the health risks associated with particular habits and behaviour, they may feel more pressure to project a laddish image in public. Some men do not like, for example, to be seen to be ordering the healthy food option when out with other men, or they may feel pressurised by male friends or colleagues at work to drink more alcohol and not to quit smoking.

Is men's health being taken more seriously?

The government first declared men's health to be an essential part of the Health of the Nation Campaign in 1992. What has been done so far to convert this political rhetoric into practical ways of communicating health education directly to men? Has the government made any difference to the funding of men's health clinics, or to the launch of men's health initiatives, such as poster and leaflet campaigns, and free telephone helplines to publicise common men's health problems in the community?

Unfortunately, there is still no added financial incentive for GPs to set up men's health clinics, except as part of their overall health promotion activities. This is in marked contrast to the provision of 'well-woman' clinics, which are financed through the additional money GPs can earn by giving out advice on family planning and taking cervical smears.

However, much has been done by the Department of Health (DoH) in terms of other men's health initiatives. For example, in response to concerns over the ever increasing number of young men being diagnosed with testicular cancer – about 1,500 new cases in the UK each year, with more than half in men under the age of 35 – the DoH produced and distributed a leaflet on testicular self-examination (a procedure described in detail on page 88).

In December 1997, the DoH launched 'CALM' (Campaign Against Living Miserably), a telephone helpline for young men having emotional or relationship problems. The pilot scheme was based in Manchester, an area where there is a particularly high number of suicides involving young men. The CALM helpline was publicised in pubs, clubs and on public transport and, following its success, there are plans to encourage other health regions to adopt a similar initiative.

In May 1998, the DoH produced a booklet called *Health Tips for Men* for men over the age of 40 which was distributed not just in GPs' surgeries but also in sports clubs and working men's clubs around the UK.

Also, in early 1998, the government published a green paper entitled *Our Healthier Nation – a Contract for Health*, which proposes a series of measures designed to address health inequalities between men and women, concentrating on four main areas: heart disease, testicular/prostate cancer, work accidents and mental health/suicide.

The Men's Health Forum, established in 1994 by the Royal College of Nursing, working in conjunction with other organisations such as the British Medical Association, is now a well-established coalition of patient groups and professional bodies, all with an interest in improving men's health. Having carried out a detailed audit of healthcare provisions for men in the UK, the Men's Health Forum now aims to carry out a number of activities to raise awareness, promote information and encourage good practice, with the objective of correcting current inequalities in men's healthcare. This group is funded by an educational grant from Merck, Sharp and Dohme, just one of several pharmaceutical companies with a commercial interest in men's health.

The Health Education Authority (HEA),* a government-funded organisation, has produced a range of men's health literature over the last few years, including:

- *Gutted*: a booklet providing advice on dealing with emotional problems, targeting mainly young men leaving home to start college or university
- *Sexual Health:* a booklet for young men

- *Healthy Living for Men*: a booklet covering diet, exercise, stress, smoking, alcohol, drugs, men's cancers, sexual health and sun safety
- *The Healthy Man's Action Pack*: including factsheets on smoking, alcohol, nutrition, physical activity, drugs, sexual health, men's cancers, skin cancer and mental health.

In addition to a few specific self-help groups, established to offer support to those men suffering from particular health disorders, such as erectile dysfunction (impotence) and prostate cancer, a new initiative entitled 'Men's Health Matters' (MHM) was launched in late 1997, with the objective of encouraging all men to seek advice about health problems sooner rather than later.

MHM runs a successful telephone advice line, staffed by a team of specially trained nurses. This service received over 1,200 calls in its first nine months, almost all the calls being from men.

Other MHM activities include the provision of factsheets on men's health topics for journalists who write in this area and, to encourage the setting up of local men's health workshops and information days, MHM is providing GP surgeries and company occupational health departments with a 'Men's Health in Practice' pack, containing practical guidelines on how to organise this type of event, along with posters, leaflets and factsheets.

Men's health and the media

And what about the media? Men's health is now beginning to receive a lot more attention on TV, radio, in magazines and newspapers but it still lags behind women's health in terms of coverage. Often it is just a single health topic that attracts all the interest.

Hot on the heels of Prozac, the antidepressant that claims to lift even the deepest depression, a great deal of hype has surrounded the launch of Viagra, the miracle cure for impotence, followed by the launch of Xenical, the wonder pill for melting away those excess pounds of flesh. Predictably, of course, a few months later, the hysteria has been replaced by the reality that, as with all new drugs, there are negatives as well as positives – that only some men will benefit from a so-called wonder drug, and that others may suffer unpleasant side-effects.

However, apart from the occasional miracle cure stories, a great deal is now being talked and written about in the media on many different men's health topics. For example, *Men's Health* magazine now has a UK circulation of just under 250,000, and a new health and fitness publication, *Zest for Men*, is due for launch at the end of 1998. In addition, all the general consumer magazines aimed at men, such as *GQ* and *Esquire* now include at least some health-related information in a format that suits their particular readership.

What this book covers

Improving men's health awareness remains a major challenge. There is still a tremendous need for widespread practical information, to guide men and their partners to better health – physical, emotional and sexual. *The Which? Guide to Men's Health* continues to bridge this health awareness and information gap.

The book was written to provide health advice and practical guidelines related specifically to the needs of men, as well as to encourage both men and their partners to take a more active interest in health issues. It shows just how easy it is for you to take control of lifestyle factors which might otherwise be undermining your physical, emotional and sexual health, without spoiling your enjoyment of life.

To help you appreciate the need to care for your body and what can go wrong with its various components, the book begins with a detailed description of the different body systems and organs. It also contains simple practical advice on how to eat better, take more exercise, give up smoking, cut down on alcohol and control stress levels.

Staying healthy is not only about having a healthy outlook, nor is this book just for those men like Harry Enfield's 'Wayne Slob', who fits the stereotype of the overweight smoker slumped in front of the TV with a can of lager and a plate of chips. It also advises on protective measures, including immunisation; it explains how to recognise the early-warning symptoms of serious illnesses (and which symptoms to report to your doctor), and how to examine different parts of your body yourself; it also tells you when to have screening tests, such as blood pressure and cholesterol measurement.

Following all this advice will not, of course, guarantee you a long life totally free from serious illness, but it will give you a much better chance of staying healthy and enjoying a better quality of life.

In this new edition is also all the latest information on Viagra and other new developments in the treatment of erectile dysfunction, along with over 50 new entries in the chapter on common health problems in men, including anorexia nervosa, Creutzfeld–Jacob disease, Klinefelter's syndrome, meningitis, panic attacks and repetitive strain injury.

As the Internet becomes an increasingly popular source of advice and information on health, the guide also includes a whole new section called 'Men's health on the Net', highlighting some of the quality web sites and also providing guidance on how to tell the difference between what is reputable and reliable and what is cranky and dubious.

Finally, I hope that, in the same way that I have learnt from my own personal experience with skin cancer, all men who read this guide will accept the challenge to take more responsibility for their own health.

Note Addresses and telephone numbers for organisations marked with an asterisk (*) can be found in the 'Addresses' section at the back of the book.

Chapter 1

Understanding the male body

IT IS NOT just doctors, nurses, other medical staff and scientists who need to know about human anatomy and physiology. Everyone should have a basic understanding of the human body and how it works. Such knowledge makes it easier for you to communicate with your doctor, easier to appreciate how an unhealthy lifestyle can damage your body, easier to come to terms with any illness or disease that affects you or someone close to you, and easier to understand why you have developed a particular symptom, why you need a specific investigation and how a drug treatment or surgical operation might help. This chapter also describes how conception occurs in women's bodies.

Heart and circulation

The heart is a powerful muscular pump which beats continuously and rhythmically to force blood into the circulation system. At rest, the normal heart rate may be as low as 50 beats per minute in some men, and as high as 90 beats per minute in others. During strenuous exercise this may increase to about 200 beats per minute.

Situated just to the left of centre of the chest, the heart is approximately the size of a clenched fist. It contains four chambers: two thin-walled upper chambers, called the atria, and two thick-walled lower chambers, called the ventricles. The heart is divided into two by a strong muscular wall, the septum, which prevents the blood flowing through the left atrium and ventricle from mixing with the blood passing through the right atrium and ventricle.

The muscle in the walls of these four chambers consists of a branching network of fibres which will go on contracting spontaneously, rhythmically and completely automatically as long as they are kept supplied with oxygen and nutrients. This type of muscle, known as the myocardium, is not found anywhere else in the body.

A smooth membrane, the endocardium, lines the inside of the heart and is continuous with the lining of the veins and arteries which feed

Figure 1: The circulation system

in and out of the heart. A tough, double-layered membranous bag, called the pericardium, surrounds and protects the heart. Between the layers of pericardium is a small amount of lubricating fluid, which allows the heart to expand freely.

How blood circulates

Blood circulates through a complex network of blood vessels in a continuous figure-of-eight circuit, with tiny branches reaching all the cells in the body to ensure they are kept supplied with blood rich in oxygen from the lungs and nutrients from the digestive system.

Oxygen-rich blood leaves the left ventricle through the aorta, which is the largest artery in the body, and is distributed to all organs and tissues through a succession of arterial branches. These arteries become smaller and smaller in diameter, until they feed into tiny vessels known as capillaries.

Oxygen, glucose (sugar) and other nutrients are absorbed into individual cells from the blood passing through nearby capillaries. Carbon dioxide and other waste products are transferred out of the cells. Having given up its oxygen and nutrients, and picked up carbon dioxide and waste products, blood passes from the capillaries into a system of veins. It is the veins that return blood to the heart. Blood returning from the stomach and intestine passes through the liver, which processes nutrients absorbed during digestion.

Two large veins, the superior (upper) vena cava and the inferior (lower) vena cava, return oxygen-depleted blood into the right atrium, from where it is passed down into the right ventricle. When the heart beats, oxygen-depleted blood leaves the right ventricle in the pulmonary artery and is pumped through the lung circulation to be replenished with oxygen. Having taken up oxygen in the lungs, blood returns to the heart in the pulmonary veins, feeding into the left atrium and then down into the left ventricle, ready for the circuit to begin again.

With each heartbeat, blood leaves both sides of the heart simultaneously so there is always some blood being reoxygenated at the same time as the rest is giving up its oxygen. Between each atrium and ventricle, and at the points where the pulmonary artery and aorta leave the heart, there are valves which prevent blood flowing in the wrong direction.

Coronary circulation

To guarantee its own blood supply, the heart has its own exclusive system of arteries, capillaries and veins, known as the coronary circulation. This begins with two arteries emerging from the start of the aorta, branching off to form three main coronary arteries.

Having supplied the heart muscle with oxygen and nutrients from the capillaries, blood is returned to the cardiac veins, which in turn drain into the right atrium.

Respiratory system

This is the system which allows you to breathe oxygen from the air into your lungs and transfer it to the circulation. At the same time, the respiratory system removes excess carbon dioxide from the blood as it passes through the lungs, allowing it to be breathed out.

Air enters the lungs through the upper respiratory tract, which consists of the nose, throat (pharynx) and voice box (larynx). These upper airways feed into the lower respiratory tract, which begins with the windpipe (trachea) and then divides into two large airways known as the bronchi.

The lungs themselves lie on either side of the heart and are cone-shaped. Air passes into each lung through one of the main bronchi, which in turn is able to carry air to and from the whole surface area of that lung by dividing into numerous small branches known as bronchioles.

At the end of each of the smallest bronchioles there are clusters of tiny balloon-like cavities known as alveoli. Over 300 million alveoli cover the entire surface of both lungs. Blood vessels running across each of the alveoli allow for efficient absorption of oxygen from the air coming in, with carbon dioxide passing in the opposite direction out of the bloodstream into the alveoli, to be breathed out.

Breathing mechanism

Breathing is a spontaneous, rhythmical, automatic activity kept going by nerve impulses transmitted from the brain stem at the base of the brain. To breathe in, the muscles between your ribs contract, pulling your rib cage upwards and outwards, and your diaphragm muscle

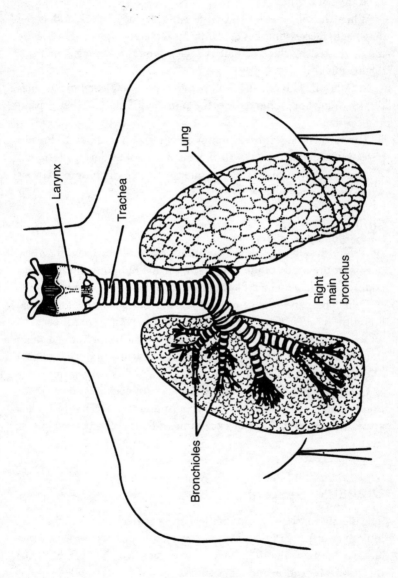

Figure 2: Respiratory system

flattens. As a result of these movements, the chest cavity around the lungs enlarges and the lungs expand to fill the extra space, sucking in air at the same time.

When the rib muscles relax, the rib cage moves back and as the diaphragm relaxes it pushes upwards. Air is thereby squeezed out of the lungs, assisted by their natural elasticity, which encourages them to shrink quickly.

In addition, a lubricating fluid between the two pleural membranes that surround both lungs reduces the amount of friction as they expand and contract.

The normal rate of breathing in an adult man is about 12 breaths per minute, reducing to 9–10 breaths per minute during sleep and increasing to over 20 breaths per minute during vigorous exercise or when under emotional stress.

Purifying the air

Breathing through the nose is healthier than mouth breathing. Not only does the inside of the nose warm up and humidify the air, it also contains tiny hairs which filter out dirt and dust particles.

Other protective mechanisms include the tiny hair-like threads (cilia) lining the insides of the trachea and bronchi, which collect particles found in polluted air, for example cigarette smoke, preventing them from entering the lungs. There is also a sticky mucus, produced by some of the cells lining the bronchi, which helps trap these impurities.

Coughing is a reflex action which can unblock the airways, for example shifting a build-up of mucus (sputum). Sneezing is a reflex action that clears particles or excess mucus from the upper respiratory tract.

Digestive system

The digestive system consists of the gastrointestinal tract – a 15-metre-long muscular organ that starts at the mouth and ends at the anus – along with several other important organs which assist with the digestion, absorption and processing of food.

In the first stage of digestion, food is ground up into smaller pieces in the mouth by the action of the teeth, tongue and the chewing muscles that pull the lower jaw upwards and move it sideways.

Figure 3: Digestive system

21

Three kinds of teeth make this process of mastication more efficient: sharp-edged cutters at the front (incisors), sharp-pointed tearers in the middle (canines) and flat-topped grinders at the back (molars and premolars).

Chewing turns food into into a paste-like mass, which the tongue then pushes towards the back of the throat. Reflex swallowing propels this food bolus down the oesophagus into the stomach, a journey that takes only two to three seconds.

Mechanical breakdown of the food continues due to churning movements of the stomach walls. Acidic gastric juices released from glands in the stomach lining begin the breakdown of proteins within the food. After two to four hours in the stomach – sometimes longer when the consumption of alcohol has delayed the reflex emptying of the stomach – partially digested food, which is now in the form of a thick liquid, passes on gradually into the small intestine.

Through the duodenum, jejunum and ileum of the small intestine the digestive processes continue, to complete the breakdown of carbohydrates, fats and proteins into molecules small enough to be absorbed through the intestinal wall. To speed up the absorption of nutrient molecules, the inside lining of the small intestine is folded into

LIVER

The liver is the largest organ in the body and is situated in the upper right area of the abdominal cavity, mostly under the lower ribs on that side. It has many different functions, among them assisting with the processing of essential nutrients:

- bile produced by the liver helps with the digestion of fats in the small intestine
- cholesterol is formed in the liver from saturated fat in the diet – some cholesterol is used to form the membranes lining new cells and to make certain hormones; too much cholesterol is bad for your heart and circulation
- surplus glucose (sugar) is converted to glycogen (starch) in the liver and stored for future energy production
- surplus amino acids from digested protein can be converted by the liver into glucose or protein.

PANCREAS

The pancreas is a gland which lies across the back wall of the abdomen, just behind and under the stomach, with one end nestling in the curve made by the duodenum and the other end situated close to the spleen.

Digestive juices produced by the pancreas and released into the duodenum contain enzymes which help complete the chemical breakdown of fats, carbohydrates and proteins. They also contain an alkali, sodium bicarbonate, which neutralises the acids that enter the duodenum from the stomach.

Hormones released by the pancreas directly into the bloodstream include insulin and glucagon, which help control the absorption of sugar from the blood into cells throughout the body.

millions of tiny projections, called villi, that massively increase the surface area in contact with the flow of digested food.

Movement of food along the small intestine is facilitated by peristalsis – continuous rhythmic contractions of the muscles in the intestinal wall. Digestion in the small intestine is aided by the action of bile, produced in the liver, stored in the gall bladder and released into the duodenum – as well as the chemical effects of several different enzymes secreted by the pancreas, also into the duodenum.

Bile assists in the digestion of fats; pancreatic enzymes break down proteins, fats and carbohydrates. The vitamins and minerals within food do not need to be digested before they can be absorbed. Within one to four hours, food will normally have reached the end of the small intestine, by which time all or most of the nutrients should have been absorbed.

Undigested matter leaving the small intestine then arrives in the last section of the gastrointestinal tract – the large intestine – which consists of the caecum, colon and rectum. Movement of the faeces (undigested matter) through the colon is again controlled by peristalsis. During the passage of faeces, most of its water and salt constituents are absorbed into the surrounding blood vessels.

The remainder of the faeces is then stored in the rectum as a semi-solid mass, ready to be expelled through the anus. Distension of the rectum by faeces is the stimulus that triggers the urge for a bowel movement.

Men appear to have a shorter transit time for the contents of their intestine than women, even when both sexes are eating the same amount of fibre in their diet. The transit time is known to vary from ten hours to as long as several days in some people, with a slower movement of faeces through the colon being associated with a greater risk of bowel cancer. This is one good reason to eat a diet high in fibre (see Chapter 2).

Kidneys and urinary system

The urinary system is designed to remove chemical waste and excess water from the body. In addition, the kidneys have a number of other important functions, including keeping the blood pressure under control.

The kidneys are a pair of bean-shaped organs surrounded by fat and situated on either side of the spine against the back wall of the abdominal cavity. Each is over 10cm long, 6cm wide and weighs nearly 0.5kg.

To fulfil its main function as an efficient filtration unit, each kidney contains around one million tiny filters known as nephrons. Each nephron starts off as a cup-shaped structure, Bowman's capsule, which surrounds a tuft of small blood vessels called the glomerulus.

Blood flowing into the glomerulus brings with it a wide range of cells and substances. Larger particles, such as red and white blood cells, platelets and blood proteins, are normally too big to filter through into the nephron. Substances consisting of smaller molecules, such as salts, glucose, minerals and chemical waste from the breakdown of worn-out cells, from muscle activity and from the processing of nutrients and drugs, are filtered from the blood into the tubule section of the nephron, along with large amounts of water.

The filtration that takes place in the glomerulus is only the first stage of the blood purification process. During its passage through the various tubule loops, the filtered liquid will lose most of its water content and controlled amounts of some of its dissolved substances back to the surrounding blood vessels. This is how the body regulates the salt and acid content of the bloodstream and keeps itself adequately hydrated.

To maintain a constant acidity level, a tight control is kept on how much acid and ammonia is taken back from the tubules. Over 80 litres

Figure 4: Kidneys and urinary system

of water filter through the kidneys every day, but about 99 per cent of this is returned from the tubules to the bloodstream. In hot weather, when more fluid is being lost from the body in sweat, the amount of water re-absorbed from the tubules will be even greater. Therefore, unless this deficit is made up by drinking larger volumes, the urine produced by the kidneys will become more concentrated.

The waste fluid left behind in each nephron's tubule empties into a funnel-shaped cavity in the centre of the kidney – the renal pelvis – from where it drains into the ureter. Each kidney has its own ureter, a narrow muscular tube about 25–30cm long that carries urine to the bladder. Constant rhythmic contraction of the muscle in the ureter wall maintains a steady urine flow. Valves in the section of the ureter within the kidney, and the diagonal position of the ureter as it passes through the bladder wall, normally prevent any backflow.

Lying behind the front section of the pelvic bone, in the mid-line, is the bladder, a muscular bag that acts as a temporary storage chamber for urine. The bladder is supported by powerful muscles in the floor of the pelvis. The urethra takes urine from the bladder along the length of the penis. A ring of muscle, known as a sphincter, surrounds the start of this narrow tube to prevent the release of urine until it is convenient.

Other kidney functions

In addition to its blood filtration and purification function, the kidney:
- activates vitamin D, which helps maintain strong, healthy bones
- produces renin, a hormone which helps to control blood pressure
- releases erythropoietin, a hormone which stimulates red blood cell production by the bone marrow.

Passing urine

As the bladder fills up, the stretching of its muscle wall sends messages to the brain that are interpreted as the desire to pass urine. Typically, this desire will disappear for a time if it is ignored, only to keep recurring at increasingly shorter intervals, until it is present constantly and too intense to ignore any longer.

When you have been drinking alcohol, you are likely to miss out the gentle early-warning signs, explaining why a visit to the toilet may suddenly become an urgent need. This is because alcohol may reduce your sensitivity to bladder impulses. It also increases the volume of urine being produced, causing the bladder to fill up more rapidly.

To urinate, the sphincter muscle around the entrance to the urethra is relaxed and as the bladder empties its muscle wall contracts to push out the urine. If the bladder is not emptied voluntarily, it will eventually empty itself spontaneously.

Endocrine system

The endocrine system consists of a collection of glands which release a variety of chemicals known as hormones into the bloodstream. Although these hormones circulate throughout the whole body, each one targets specific tissues or organs which are programmed to respond to it.

Many different aspects of physical and mental function are activated and controlled by hormones, including growth, sexual development, response to stress and cell metabolism (energy-producing and -consuming processes). The greater the concentration of a particular hormone which is circulating in the blood, the stronger its effects will be, assuming the target tissues and organs are responding normally.

To understand how the endocrine system works, it is easiest to consider each component in turn, starting with the two control centres in the brain. The hypothalamus, situated on the underside of the brain, exerts overall control of the endocrine system. Activity in the pituitary gland (see below) is influenced by both nerve impulses and by a selection of hormones released from the hypothalamus. Psychological stimuli, such as fear, anger or sexual arousal, are able to trigger physical changes in the body by altering activity in the hypothalamus, which in turn influences the production and release of different hormones by the pituitary and other glands.

The pituitary gland, also located at the base of the brain and connected to the hypothalamus by a short stalk, produces a variety of its own hormones, as well as controlling hormone production by other endocrine glands. Pituitary hormones include:

- growth hormone, which regulates body growth and development
- antidiuretic hormone, which increases water reabsorption from the kidney tubules
- thyroid stimulating hormone (TSH), which maintains consistent production of thyroid hormones by the thyroid gland
- adrenocorticotrophic hormone (ACTH), which maintains consistent production of cortisol by the adrenal glands.

Thyroid gland

Hormones produced by the thyroid gland stimulate metabolism in nearly every cell in the body and help maintain body temperature. Situated at the front of the neck, the thyroid gland also assists the control of calcium levels in the blood through the action of an additional hormone called calcitonin.

The small parathyroid glands, situated within the thyroid gland, produce parathyroid hormone, which has the opposite effect to calcitonin on blood calcium levels. If the concentration of calcium in the blood is too low, an increased output of parathyroid hormone restores the calcium level to normal.

Pancreas

In addition to its production of digestive enzymes (see page 23), the pancreas releases two hormones into the bloodstream – insulin and glucagon – which together control the concentration of glucose (sugar) in the blood.

Adrenal glands

This pair of small, triangular glands fits like a cap on top of each kidney. Hormones produced by the adrenal glands include:

- aldosterone, which is released in response to the action of renin from the kidney to control the body's salt and water balance
- cortisol (hydrocortisone), which is released in response to the action of ACTH from the pituitary gland to control the body's use of carbohydrates, fats and proteins; it also suppresses excessive inflammatory reactions and assists recovery from injury, illness or surgery
- adrenaline, which is released in response to nerve stimulation from the hypothalamus as a reaction to stress, fear or excitement. The

actions of adrenaline are the basis of the primitive 'fight or flight' response (see also page 31) and include a faster rate of breathing and more rapid pulse

- androgens, which are continuously released in small amounts from the adrenal glands and, along with androgens produced by the testicles, are important in the development and maintenance of strong healthy bones and muscles.

Testicles

Specialised cells in the testicles produce several androgen hormones, the most potent of which is testosterone, in response to the release of gonadotrophin hormones from the pituitary gland. Androgens from the testicles are more active than adrenal gland androgens; they stimulate the appearance of male sexual characteristics at puberty, including enlargement of the penis, growth of facial and body hair, and increased bulk of the muscles, particularly around the chest and shoulders. Testicular androgens, like the adrenal androgens, also stimulate bone and muscle growth.

Brain and nervous system

The brain is the control centre of the body. At all times, even during sleep, the brain receives, sorts, interprets and stores information transmitted as nerve impulses from every part of the body.

Some of this sensory information results in conscious awareness of an outside event or internal change in the body. The brain may then initiate a controlled movement in response to this sensation. However, a lot of the incoming data simply triggers an automatic or reflex adjustment, such as a change in posture or alteration in blood flow, of which the individual is not aware.

The brain is also the seat of emotion, instinct and intellect. It is the memory store which records experiences and enables the individual to learn. The brain determines personality, behaviour, creativity and talent for physical and mental tasks.

Brain structure

Weighing over 1kg and containing over 100 billion nerve cells, the brain occupies most of the space inside the skull. In addition to the skull's bony protection, a layer of cerebrospinal fluid (CSF) between two of the three outer brain membranes (meninges) provides extra cushioning to reduce the risk of damage to the sensitive nerve cells.

The largest section of the brain is the cerebrum, which is divided into two almost identical hemispheres connected by a large bundle of nerve fibres called the corpus callosum. The thin outer surface of these hemispheres – the cerebral cortex – is folded into a number of different lobes, separated by deep clefts and named after the skull bones that lie directly over them: frontal, temporal, parietal and occipital lobes.

In only a few areas of the cerebral cortex have specific functions, such as initiating movement, responding to visual images, or understanding language, been identified.

Beneath the six layers of nerve cells that make up the cerebral cortex (the so-called grey matter), much of the remainder of the cerebrum consists of nerve tracts (the white matter), which connect various areas of the cortex together. These tracts are also linked to a number of important nerve centres deeper within the brain, including:

- the hypothalamus, which helps control appetite, thirst and body temperature and influences sleep, aggression and sexual behaviour
- the pituitary gland, which produces a variety of hormones and controls other endocrine glands (see page 27)
- the limbic system, which handles emotions, processes smell sensations and is involved in registration and recall of memories
- the cerebellum, which is concerned with balance, muscle co-ordination and posture.
- the basal ganglia, which control complex body movements through connections to the cerebellum

Brain stem and spinal cord

Just in front of the cerebellum, passing downwards from the middle of the underside of the cerebrum, is a thick stalk which carries major nerve tracts running between the brain and spinal cord, and *vice versa*. Inside this brain stem are the nerve centres which control heartbeat and breathing.

Below the brain stem, the spinal cord runs down through a large hole in the base of the skull and passes on down a canal in the centre of the spinal column. The brain and spinal cord together form the central nervous system (CNS). Nerves from the peripheral nervous system run into and out of the spinal cord between adjacent pairs of vertebrae.

Peripheral nervous system

This part of the nervous system consists of sensory nerves, which carry information from all areas of the body to the CNS, along with motor nerves, which take instructions from the CNS out to individual groups of muscles to initiate movement.

Nerve impulses arriving from sensory nerve fibres may be carried up the spinal cord and brain stem into the part of the cerebral cortex designed to analyse and interpret them. The brain may then initiate a response which passes as nerve impulses down through the brain stem and spinal cord, emerging along specific motor nerve fibres to cause a particular muscle to contract.

Because the nerve tracts cross, movement of the right-hand side of the body is controlled by the left side of the brain, and the left-hand side by the right side of the brain.

Muscles normally controlled by the brain may also respond as an automatic reflex, for example, in reaction to a painful stimulus. In this situation, the sensory signal that reaches the spinal cord makes direct contact with the motor nerve nearby, without having to pass up to the brain first. Reflexes are important as a protective mechanism: for example, they make it possible for you to pull your hand quickly away from something that is hot enough to cause a burn.

The brain, however, can override a reflex, for example allowing you to walk across burning ashes, or consciously suppressing contraction of the muscles on the front of the thigh when a doctor tests the knee-jerk reflex.

Autonomic nervous system

This part of the nervous system is concerned with body functions that work without conscious control. Autonomic nerves regulate blood pressure, sweating, skin blood flow, sexual arousal, including erection and ejaculation, body temperature and the passage of intestinal contents by peristalsis.

The autonomic nervous system is divided into sympathetic nerves, which trigger the 'fight or flight' response to dangerous or frightening situations, and parasympathetic nerves which are primarily involved in body functions at rest or asleep.

Most of the autonomic nerve cells run parallel to the spine as a chain of linked clumps known as ganglia, with autonomic fibres passing along the same routes as some of the nerves from the peripheral nervous system.

Eyes

The eye is a fluid-filled ball, roughly spherical in shape, that is held inside a bony socket in the skull by three pairs of muscles, which also control its movement.

Most of the focusing in the eye is done by the cornea, the front part of the tough outer coating of the eye, which is transparent and shaped like a dome. Light passes through the cornea and then on through a hole in the centre of the iris, known as the pupil.

Additional focusing is done by the lens in each eye. This elastic, transparent structure is suspended within a circular ring of muscle, known as the ciliary body. Contraction or relaxation of this muscle changes the shape of the lens, allowing the eye to focus on a particular object by accurately directing all the light rays to cross each other on the surface of the retina at the back of the eye.

The amount of light entering the eye is controlled by the action of muscle fibres within the iris. In dark conditions, radial fibres contract as a reflex to widen the pupil and let more light in. When there is bright light, circular fibres contract to narrow the pupil.

Visualising an image

Millions of light-sensitive cells in the retina – rods and cones – convert the light rays they come into contact with into nerve impulses, which are then transferred to the brain along the optic nerve. Rods are concerned with the fine detail of an image, cones are each sensitive to one of the three primary colours: red, blue or yellow.

The image formed on the retina is actually upside down, but as part of its ability to interpret the nerve impulses it receives from each eye, the brain learns to turn the picture the correct way up. Images are assembled in the visual cortex at the back of the brain.

Crossover of some of the optic nerve fibres behind the eyes means that both sides of the brain receive signals from both eyes. Because the images from the two eyes differ slightly, the brain is able to produce a

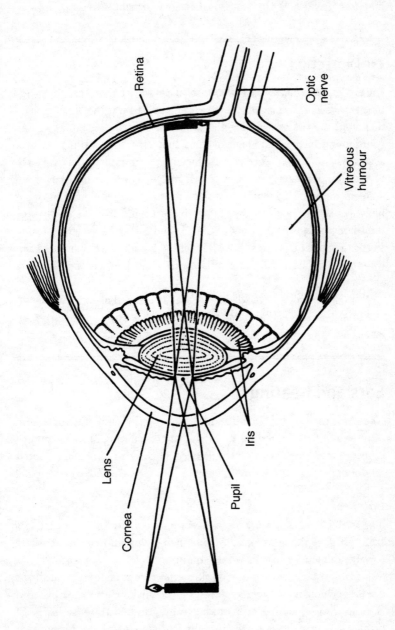

Figure 5: Eye structure

three-dimensional view of its surroundings, judging depth as well as height and width. Two eyes also offer a wider field of vision.

EYE PROTECTION

The eyelids close quickly as a reflex mechanism when any object approaches the eye. A row of tiny glands on each eyelid produces small amounts of an oil that stops the lids sticking together when the eyes are closed, as well as contributing to the thin sheet of tears that constantly bathes the eye. Eyelashes are strong, curved hairs arranged in two rows along the front edge of each eyelid. They trap particles of dust and grit blown into the eye.

Tears are produced by glands inside the upper and outer margins of the bony eye socket and also by glands in the conjunctiva, a thin layer of transparent skin over the front of the eye and under the eyelids. Blinking sweeps a film of tears across the eye, keeping its surface well lubricated and washing away dust and dirt. In addition to salty water, tears contain a natural antiseptic.

Tears drain through a single hole near the inner end of each eyelid, first into small tear sacs and then into the nose, which is why your nose may run if you cry.

Ears and hearing

The ear is designed to pick up sound waves – rhythmic, rapid pressure changes in the surrounding air produced by vibrating objects – and to convert these sound waves into electrical signals that can be interpreted by the brain. There are three main sections to each ear.

Outer ear

The visible part of the ear, known as the pinna, consists of a cartilage skeleton covered with skin. Although it helps funnel sound waves towards the eardrum, you would still be able to hear without it.

Sound then passes along a skin-lined passage – the auditory canal – which is about 2cm long, before striking the eardrum and causing it to vibrate. Wax is produced by glands within the lining of this canal, normally in small amounts that clear naturally. Along with the hairs at the entrance to the ear, the wax traps dirt and dust particles.

Semi-circular canal

Stapes (stirrup)

Cochlea

Skull bone

Eustachian tube

Incus (anvil)

Malleus (hammer)

Tympanic membrane (eardrum)

Outer ear canal

Pinna

Figure 6: Ear structure

The eardrum is a delicate membrane that separates the outer and middle ear; when healthy it vibrates in sympathy with the incoming sound waves.

Middle ear

This small air-filled cavity is crossed by three tiny, moveable and inter-linked bones (the hammer, anvil and stirrup). Vibrations of the eardrum are amplified as they are transmitted across these bones to a window in the outside wall of the inner ear.

To keep the air pressure inside the middle ear equal to the air pressure against the outside of the eardrum, and thereby allow the eardrum to vibrate freely, the middle ear cavity is connected to the back of the throat by the eustachian tube.

Inner ear

The hearing part of the inner ear, the cochlea, consists of a spiral membrane, known as the basilar membrane, bathed in fluid that starts to vibrate in response to incoming vibrations from the middle ear. The spiral structure of the cochlea resembles a small snail shell.

Different sections of the membrane vibrate according to the exact frequency of the pressure waves. Hair cells lining the vibrating part of the membrane are also set in motion and because each of these hairs is connected to a nerve fibre the vibration is converted into an electrical impulse.

A pattern of electrical impulses, corresponding to the incoming pattern of sound waves, is then conveyed to the brain along the auditory nerve. In the part of the brain where these signals are processed – the auditory cortex – they are interpreted as a particular sound on the basis of previous experiences of sound held in the memory.

Finally, at the back of the inner ear, three fluid-filled semi-circular canals at right angles to each other help to maintain balance by detecting even the slightest body movement.

Smell, taste and touch

Smell

Microscopic chemical particles carried in the air are detected as a particular smell by sensitive hair-like nerve endings lining the roof of the nose. These odorous molecules become trapped in the secretions produced by the mucous lining of the nose and when they come into contact with the olfactory nerve filaments, electrical impulses are relayed to the base of the brain. Different types of particle relating to different odours stimulate their own unique pattern of nerve impulses, which can then be interpreted by the brain on the basis of previous experience.

Taste

About 10,000 taste buds are positioned on the top and sides of the tongue, as well as being scattered over the roof and back of the mouth. There are four main taste sensations: sweetness, detected by taste buds at the tip of the tongue; bitterness, by those at the back of the tongue; sourness, by those in the middle of the tongue sides; and saltiness by taste buds at the front of the tongue sides.

Chemicals in food or drink dissolve in saliva and then penetrate pores in the tongue surface to reach the underlying taste buds. Stimulation of a taste bud triggers an electrical impulse in the attached nerve fibre, which is transmitted to the brain for interpretation.

Although the taste buds can only distinguish the four basic tastes, a wide range of flavours can be appreciated through the involvement of smell receptors in the nose. These receptors are stimulated by food odours passing up from the back of the throat, which is why anyone with a nose blocked by mucus due to a cold is likely to experience a marked loss of taste.

Touch

Buried in the skin are many types of sensory receptors which respond to different forms of external stimulation, such as fine touch, pressure, pain, heat and cold. Some of these receptors are just a single nerve fibre wrapped around an individual hair so that it can respond to any movement of that hair. Others are more complex, containing several layers of cells, with nerve fibres arranged in a loop or coil.

Signals are carried from these receptors along sensory nerves to the spinal cord (see page 30) and on up to the area of the brain, known as the sensory cortex, where different skin sensations are processed and interpreted.

Some areas of skin are more sensitive to painful stimuli, or better able to discriminate between close points of touch, because they contain a greater number of the appropriate receptors. Also, the most sensitive parts of the body, including the hands, feet, lips and genitals, are represented by larger areas of the sensory cortex in the brain.

Skin, hair and nails

Skin

The skin does a lot more than just hold the organs and fluids of the body together. This complex structure, which itself is one of the body's largest organs, weighing over 4kg and covering a total area of over 2 square metres, performs the following different functions:

- stops body tissue absorbing water like a sponge, while retaining enough moisture to stay supple
- keeps out bacteria and chemicals
- uses the sun's ultraviolet rays to manufacture vitamin D
- responds to pain, touch, temperature and pressure, sending this information to the brain for processing and interpretation
- controls body temperature.

Epidermal layer

The epidermis is the thin outer layer of skin. On its surface, there are layers of flat dead cells which contain a type of protein known as keratin. This is what provides the skin with its tough, waterproof protective coating.

The dead skin cells are continuously being discarded, particularly when you wash or dry your body. Areas of the body that experience the most wear and tear, such as the palms and soles, develop a thicker layer of these protective cells.

To replace the outer skin cells, new, living epidermal cells are continuously produced underneath them. It normally takes about four weeks for the new cells to migrate to the skin surface, dying on the way up.

Special skin cells called melanocytes produce the pigment melanin that helps shield the body from the sun's ultraviolet rays and gives the skin its colour. The degree of pigmentation depends on the number and activity of these melanocytes, which is primarily genetically determined. Melanin production can be stimulated by regular sun exposure to produce a tan.

Dermal layer

Much thicker than the epidermis, the dermis contains connective tissues which give the skin both resilience and elasticity. Embedded within this connective tissue are a variety of specialised structures, including sweat and sebaceous (oil-producing) glands, sensory receptors and hair follicles. There is also a network of tiny blood vessels to keep the cells supplied with oxygen and nutrients.

Subcutaneous layer

Below the dermis is a layer of subcutaneous fat, which varies in thickness around the body. These fat cells can act as a source of reserve fuel and also provide protection and insulation for internal body organs.

Hair function and growth

Hair is basically composed of dead cells plus keratin, the protein also found in skin. Each shaft of hair consists of a spongy semi-hollow core (the medulla), made of soft rectangular cells; a surrounding layer of long, thin fibres (the cortex), made of cells which become harder as they emerge from the scalp or skin; and an outer layer of overlapping, flat cells (the cuticle) arranged like slates on a roof.

The root of each hair is firmly enclosed by a cluster of living cells at the base of the hair follicle, known as the bulb, which produce keratin while the hair is actively growing. Within the bulb is a mass of cells – the papilla – and nerve endings, which explains why pulling out a hair is painful.

Each hair grows for a period lasting between two and five years, before entering the so-called resting phase. As growth stops, the bulb pulls back from the hair root and the hair falls out. After about three months, a new hair begins to grow, to take its place.

Different hairs enter this resting phase at different times, resulting in a variable loss of scalp hair of anything between 50 and 150 hairs each day.

The pigment melanin gives hair its colour. Red or auburn hair results from varying amounts of the red type of melanin; colours ranging from black to blonde depend on the proportion of the brown type of melanin. Hair turns white or grey when the production of melanin ceases.

Nails

Not only do nails protect the tips of the fingers and toes, they also assist in the manipulation of objects and provide a useful tool for scratching.

Each nail consists of a hard curved plate made of keratin, the same protein that is found in skin and hair. The base of the nail plate is paler than the rest of it and shaped like a half moon; overlying this area of nail is a flap of free skin known as the cuticle.

Under the nail plate, at the base of the nail bed, is the area of tissue from which the nail grows. Fingernails normally grow at a rate of about 1cm every three months, so it takes up to five months to grow a completely new nail on the finger. Toenails grow at least twice as slowly, which is why you don't have to cut them so often.

Bones and joints

Bone consists of a tough, rubbery protein called collagen, which is impregnated with the minerals calcium and phosphorus to make it rigid. The resultant structure is light, but incredibly strong.

An outer, hard layer, known as cortical bone, surrounds a spongy core which contains the liquid bone marrow. While the shafts of the long bones are mainly hollow, the ends are filled with this spongy type of bone, arranged in struts to provide added strength.

A dense membrane, the periosteum, lines the outside of all bones. Blood vessels running in the periosteum and through canals in the cortical bone keep the bone tissue alive by supplying nutrients and oxygen. They also take away the new blood cells being continuously produced by the bone marrow (see page 45).

A total of 206 bones usually makes up the framework of an adult skeleton, although some people have an extra pair of ribs, or an additional bone in their hands or feet. There are no major differences between the skeleton of a man and a woman. However, bones are usually larger and heavier in men and the pelvis narrower.

In addition to providing a supporting structure and anchorage for the skeletal muscles, bone has several other important functions:

- protection of delicate internal organs, such as the brain and heart
- blood cell production in bone marrow, mainly within flat bones such as the pelvis, ribs, sternum and skull
- supply of calcium into the bloodstream when required.

Bone growth and healing

As a child grows, new bone is formed from cartilage plates that lie across the shaft, near each end of the long bones. Cartilage is changed into bone on the side of this epiphyseal plate nearest the centre of the bone, but the thickness of the plate remains the same as new cartilage is formed on its outer surface. These changes are stimulated by the action of growth hormone, causing the bones to lengthen.

Growth ceases in early adult life when the epiphyseal plates are entirely converted into bone. However, the two types of bone cell which are involved in the formation of new bone – osteoblasts and osteoclasts – continue to function within the bones, to keep their internal structure strong and healthy.

After a fracture, the osteoblasts and osteoclasts assist the repair process. Osteoblasts lay down new collagen within the blood clot that forms between the broken ends. Osteoclasts remove unwanted bone debris and release minerals which can be re-used in the formation of new bone.

Bone tissues are alive: new bone forms and old bone degenerates throughout life. This activity slows down with advancing years, which explains why older men have weaker bones that are more likely to fracture.

Various hormones control bone metabolism in men, including testosterone, adrenal hormones, parathyroid hormone and growth hormone. As there is no major change in any of these controlling hormones with ageing, men are less vulnerable to osteoporosis than women, who at the menopause gradually lose the beneficial action of the female sex hormone oestrogen on their bones.

Joint structure and movement

Joints are the junctions where bones meet. Not all joints move – there are fixed joints in the skull which fuse in childhood once the head has stopped growing.

In a mobile joint, the ends where the bones meet have a protective covering of cartilage, which provides a smooth, low-friction but hard-wearing surface. A fibrous capsule surrounds and protects the joint, and inside this capsule some joints have a thin synovial membrane which releases small amounts of fluid. This synovial fluid acts as a joint lubricant, as well as keeping the internal cartilage surfaces supplied with oxygen and nutrients.

A joint moves as a result of either the contraction of muscles that pass across it, or the pull of a tendon on one of the bones. Although the amount of movement in each different direction is determined primarily by the shape of the internal joint surfaces, tough bands of elastic tissue called ligaments normally prevent overstretching of a joint.

The main types of joint, each with their own characteristic range of movements, are:

- ball and socket joints, which allow movement of one bone in all directions; e.g. shoulder, hip
- hinge joints, which move in one plane only; e.g. elbow (the knee is not just a hinge joint, as it also allows the lower leg to rotate)
- pivot joints, which allow rotation only; e.g. joint between upper two neck bones
- gliding joints, which allow movement between two almost flat or slightly curved surfaces; e.g. spinal joints
- ellipsoidal joints, which consist of an oval protrusion fitting into an oval hollow, allowing all movements except rotation; e.g. wrist joint
- saddle joints, where the surfaces curve outward in one direction and inward in the other; e.g. the joint at the base of the thumb
- fixed joints, skull suture joints allow no movement in adults; sacroiliac joints on either side of the back of the pelvis permit only slight movement.

Skeletal muscles

Skeletal muscles are attached to the bones, either directly or via tendons formed from the outer muscle sheath. They maintain body posture and generate movements of the head, trunk and limbs.

Skeletal muscles are under conscious control (see 'Peripheral nervous system', page 31). Stimulation of a muscle by its incoming motor nerve causes the fibres within it to contract. This contraction involves the sliding movement of specialised proteins, arranged as parallel overlapping rods inside the hundreds of long filaments that make up each muscle fibre. The muscle fibres are shortened in proportion to the amount of overlap.

Figure 7: Examples of joints in the body

To move a particular part of the body, usually one group of skeletal muscles is contracted while the group with the opposite action is relaxed. Muscles are broadly classified according to the type of movement they perform: for example, adductors move part of the body inwards, abductors move it outwards, levators raise it and depressors lower it. Extensor muscles open a joint, flexors close it.

Cardiac and smooth muscle

These other two types of muscle in the body are controlled unconsciously by the autonomic nervous system (see page 31). Contraction and relaxation of these muscles change the shape or volume of internal structures, such as organs and blood vessels.

Cardiac muscle (the myocardium), which makes up the walls of the four heart chambers, is designed to continuously pump blood out into the circulation. Smooth muscle is arranged in circular bands around blood vessels to control their diameter and thus the flow of blood. The intestine has smooth muscle fibres around its circumference as well as along the length of the wall. Regular contraction and relaxation of these muscle bands produces a movement known as peristalsis, which squeezes the intestinal contents forwards.

Blood and lymph

In an adult man, about six litres of blood flow through the circulation system. Just over half of this volume is a pale, amber substance known as plasma, 90 per cent of which is water in which a wide variety of constituents are dissolved, including various salts, nutrients, enzymes, antibodies and blood-clotting proteins. The remaining 45 or so per cent of the blood volume is made up of red blood cells, platelets and white blood cells. The purpose of blood is:

- to carry oxygen and nutrients to every cell in the body
- to remove carbon dioxide and other waste products from tissues (for elimination through the lungs and kidneys)
- to seal up any damage to a blood vessel, through the formation of a blood clot
- to provide a highly mobile defence system against invading organisms.

Red blood cells

These flat, disc-shaped cells are constantly being made in the bone marrow, from where they are fed into the bloodstream. They carry oxygen into the tissues, where they exchange it for carbon dioxide which they then return to the lungs. Haemoglobin, a pigment made from iron, is the component of the red blood cell designed to gather and release oxygen. There are about five million red blood cells per cubic millimetre of blood.

Platelets

These round, flattened particles, also produced in the bone marrow, are the smallest type of blood cell in the circulation. There are about 250,000 platelets per cubic millimetre of blood.

Platelets play a key role in the process of blood clotting. In contact with a damaged vessel wall, the platelets become chemically activated and, as a result, start to clump together to plug the hole. Activated platelets also release chemicals that stimulate the formation of fibrin from other blood-clotting substances which are being carried in the plasma.

Filaments of fibrin combine with clumps of platelets and also with red and white blood cells to form a solid blood clot. The sealing of damaged blood vessels with a clot helps to keep the amount of blood lost from the circulation to a minimum.

White blood cells

Several different types of white blood cell are found in the circulation, together totalling about 7,500 per cubic millimetre of blood. White blood cells are also made in the bone marrow, but they mature in several other tissues in the body, including the lymph nodes, the spleen, tonsils and the thymus, which is a gland situated behind the breast bone.

The lifespan of a white blood cell is highly variable. Some may last for many years, others for only a few hours. During an infection, millions of white cells may be destroyed while dealing with the invading bugs.

Unlike red blood cells, which are confined to the bloodstream, white blood cells are able to push their way through the walls of both blood and lymph vessels (see 'Lymphatic system' overleaf), thereby reaching the site of an infection, tumour or injury.

Varieties of white blood cell include:

- neutrophils, which directly attack and engulf invading bugs, often with the formation of pus consisting of dead neutrophils and bacteria
- basophils, which release chemicals that trigger allergic and inflammatory reactions
- eosinophils, which proliferate in response to allergic reactions or parasite infections
- monocytes, which can enlarge to become macrophages that penetrate infected tissue and, like neutrophils, engulf and kill bacteria and other organisms
- lymphocytes, which can target, neutralise and destroy foreign cells, including bugs, tumour cells and substances that provoke an allergic reaction.

BLOOD GROUPS

Red blood cells in the circulation carry certain types of protein on their surface called antigens. Everyone's blood can be classified into a particular blood group, based on the presence or absence of antigens. The main antigens are those from the ABO system, along with the rhesus antigen, to produce four basic blood groups: AB, A, B and O, all either rhesus positive or rhesus negative. Before a blood transfusion, the doctor will check that the donated blood is compatible with the patient's blood group to avoid an unpleasant, potentially fatal, reaction.

Lymphatic system

The thin-walled transparent vessels that make up the lymphatic system start as blind-ended capillaries, which penetrate most body tissues. These lymph capillaries drain into larger lymphatic vessels, which have internal valves to ensure there is no backflow.

Lymph, a clear, protein-rich fluid, passes towards the heart through this network of vessels, driven by pressure from the contraction of surrounding muscles together with the constant pressure changes inside the abdominal and chest cavities. The majority of lymph vessels run alongside the arteries and veins of the blood circulation.

Scattered throughout the body are bean-shaped lymph nodes, each of which receives lymph from one or more lymphatic vessels and drains it into at least one exit vessel. These lymph nodes are located under the arms, in the groins and around the neck, as well as deep in the chest and abdomen. There is also a similar type of lymph tissue, situated inside the liver and spleen.

Having passed through these lymph nodes, lymph drains through to the upper part of the chest, emptying ultimately into the bloodstream through the large veins at the base of the neck.

The three main functions of the lymphatic system are:

- to absorb digested fats from the small intestine
- to collect up protein and water that the blood circulation has left behind in the tissues
- to assist the body's immune system (see below).

Immune system

To protect the body from the millions of harmful bugs, chemicals and other substances that bombard it over a lifetime, there is a complex network of natural defences known as the immune system. The main task of the immune system is to neutralise and destroy bugs, such as bacteria or viruses, which could otherwise seriously damage body organs or tissues, either by infecting them or by releasing toxins that poison their cells.

The first line of defence consists of various physical and chemical barriers to infection, which together are classified as the body's innate immune system. These different barriers include:

- antiseptic substances present in saliva, tears and sweat
- acids in the stomach, which kill most bugs
- friendly bacteria in the intestine and on the skin, which restrict the growth of harmful bugs
- mucus in the nose and other airways, which traps bugs and is then either swallowed, sneezed or coughed up.

Any bug or foreign substance that bypasses the innate immune system is immediately attacked by white blood cells – the adaptive immune system. These cells can destroy invaders by means of several different mechanisms:

- some lymphocytes produce antibodies, which latch on to one of the surface proteins (antigens) of the invaders, either killing them, or making it easier for other white blood cells to devour them
- other lymphocytes, which are able to target the invader directly, may multiply rapidly and then attack the invading bugs or offending tumour cells
- certain white blood cells, like eosinophils and basophils, deal with a foreign cell or substance by releasing chemicals that assist the function of the lymphocytes and macrophages.

In addition to circulating in the bloodstream, lymphocytes congregate in the lymph nodes ready to deal with bugs that have been drawn into the lymphatic system from surrounding tissues. In this way an infection may be kept localised, instead of spreading to the rest of the body, which is why, for example, an infected finger may cause tender, swollen lymph nodes under the arm. Lymph tissue in the liver and spleen is designed to filter out and destroy bugs being carried in the bloodstream.

Immunity

Immunity is the ability to recognise an invading bug previously encountered, allowing the immune system to respond rapidly to any subsequent attack before the infection has time to take hold. This phenomenon is the result of the formation of a 'memory' cell from one type of lymphocyte, which carries an exact blueprint of the invader's distinguishing antigen.

Immunisation is the exposure of the body to a weakened or dead strain of a particular type of bug, which artificially stimulates immunity to that infection (see pages 93–4).

Male reproductive system

The male reproductive system has three main functions: the production and storage of sperm; the production and release of sperm-containing seminal fluid during ejaculation; and the production of the male sex hormone testosterone.

While most men are aware of the basic anatomy of their genitals, certainly of the visible parts, there is a great deal of ignorance about what goes on beneath the surface. Understanding the position and function of structures like the prostate gland and the vas deferens will

Figure 8: Male reproductive system

be useful, for example, if you ever have problems with an enlarged prostate, or you are going to have a vasectomy (see pages 135–8).

Penis

Inside the penis are three cylinders of spongy tissue, two on the upper side, known as the corpora cavernosa, and one on the underside, the corpus spongiosum. When the penis is flaccid these three chambers are squashed flat; sexual stimulation causes the corpora cavernosa to become engorged with blood through a network of blood vessels, resulting in an erection.

Down through the corpus spongiosum runs the urethra, which is a muscular tube about 25cm long that carries urine and semen to the tip of the penis. The glans, the head of the penis, which is the end of the corpus spongiosum, is covered in uncircumcised men by a loose fold of skin called the prepuce or foreskin.

Testicles

These two sex glands, the male equivalent of the female's ovaries, manufacture sperm and the sex hormone testosterone. They hang together, but at different heights, within a wrinkled pouch of skin known as the scrotum, which is located below and behind the penis.

There is a good reason for positioning the testicles within the scrotum rather than inside the abdomen. The circulation of air around the scrotum keeps the testicles at a temperature around 5°C lower than the normal body temperature. This appears to enhance both sperm production and the release of testosterone.

Within each testicle are about 1,000 tiny tubes, coiled up like spaghetti. Unravelled and laid end to end, these would span a length of nearly 500 metres. Cells inside these seminiferous tubules start to produce immature sperm from puberty onwards, with each sperm then taking about ten weeks to become fully developed. All the seminiferous tubules feed into the epididymis, which is a tightly coiled tube lying behind the testicle. In the epididymis, the sperm are stored and continue to mature over two to three weeks, after which they are ready to be ejaculated. As many as 500 million mature sperm reach the end of the epididymis each day.

A mature sperm cell is only about 0.05mm long and consists of a head, neck, midpiece, tail and endpiece. Healthy sperm have an oval-shaped head, which contains the genetic material that the father will contribute to his child should conception take place. The rest of the sperm is designed solely to generate the whip-like movements of the tail that propel it along.

Testosterone, a natural anabolic steroid hormone, is produced by specialised cells, known as Leydig cells, scattered between the lines of seminiferous tubules within each testicle. The production of testosterone by the testicles increases at puberty to cause the characteristic physical changes (see page 57).

Vas deferens

Prior to ejaculation, sperm are transported from the epididymis through a long duct, the vas deferens, towards the entrance to the urethra. About 60 per cent of the seminal fluid produced during ejaculation is released by the seminal vesicles into the vas deferens, to join the sperm on the way to the urethra.

Prostate

The prostate gland, which is normally the size of a chestnut in the adult male, is situated at the base of the bladder and surrounds the urethra. Secretions produced by the prostate are added to the seminal fluid while it is collecting at the start of the urethra, a few seconds before ejaculation occurs.

SEMEN

This thick, milky fluid, produced by the seminal vesicles and prostate gland, is added to sperm before ejaculation to provide nourishment for the millions of sperm cells. In the average man, the volume of semen released in one ejaculation is one teaspoonful or less.

Although about 90 per cent of semen is water, it contains a variety of essential nutrients, including zinc, potassium, glucose and vitamin C, which keep the ejaculated sperm alive and kicking.

Sexual arousal and responses

A wide variety of stimuli can sexually excite a man, causing a burst of electrical impulses from nerve centres close to the spinal cord, which produces an erection. This reflex response is controlled by other nerve centres in the brain, which react positively to erotic sensations. It may also be suppressed by feelings such as anxiety and guilt, leading to loss of erection or failure to get an erection in the first place.

Different men respond to different erotic stimuli. Men are said to be more responsive to visual eroticism than women, but it is always dangerous to make these sorts of generalisations. A vital part of any sexual relationship is discovering what turns you on and letting your partner know how to get you aroused – and *vice versa*, of course.

Erections may also occur spontaneously during the dreaming phases of sleep and men commonly wake with an erection in the morning, although, more often than not, there will be no recollection of an erotic dream.

Two American experts in human sexuality, Masters and Johnson, were the first to produce (in 1966) a detailed description of the various phases of sexual response in men.

Excitation phase   The first stage of sexual arousal, the development of an erection, is the result of engorgement of the penis with blood, causing its spongy tissues to increase in length and volume and the overlying skin to stretch taut. An erection may come on within a few seconds or build up gradually, depending on the individual and the intensity of arousal. Muscles at the base of the penis are also stimulated to contract, maintaining the erection by preventing blood from escaping.

Plateau phase   The name of this, the second stage of sexual arousal, is misleading because it actually involves a progressive increase in sexual tension. In addition to the penis becoming erect, the lower part of the glans swells and the testicles enlarge to one-and-a-half times their resting size as a result of becoming engorged with blood. The testicles are also pulled upwards closer to the body.

The man's skin may start to flush red and usually his pulse, blood pressure and breathing rate will increase, owing to nerve activation rather than exertion. A few drops of clear, sticky fluid may seep out of the urethra at the tip of the penis, to lubricate the foreskin (if there is one) and neutralise any traces of urine that might otherwise harm the sperm about to be ejaculated. Because these secretions (which come from the Cowper's glands under the prostate) may occasionally contain sperm, there is a risk that pregnancy may result from unprotected intercourse with a woman, even without ejaculation.

Emission phase If sexual stimulation continues for long enough during the plateau phase, preparation for ejaculation begins with an emission phase that lasts just a few seconds and from which there is no turning back. Contraction of the seminal vesicles massages semen into the vas deferens to join the sperm moving towards the start of the urethra. As sperm and semen arrive in the urethra, it stretches to accommodate this fluid and contraction of the prostate gland adds further seminal secretions.

Muscles at the entrance to the urethra from the bladder are normally tightly contracted at this stage to prevent semen escaping backwards, and urine from being passed out during ejaculation.

Orgasm phase The muscles which surround the urethra and support the base of the penis begin to contract rhythmically and regularly. Seminal fluid is forced along the urethra and pumped out of the tip of the penis under pressure. Usually the semen spurts out, although sometimes – particularly in older men or men ejaculating for a second time in quick succession – it may just ooze.

In addition to the ejaculation of semen, powerful reflex contractions of muscles in the abdomen, pelvis and buttocks all contribute to the overall sensation of orgasm.

Resolution phase For the first few seconds after ejaculation, the glans becomes extremely sensitive and continued stimulation may even be painful. Usually, there is an almost immediate loss of erection, with the penis rapidly returning to half its erect size, before slowly shrinking back to its non-aroused condition. The testicles also decrease to their resting size and are lowered to their normal position.

A pleasant feeling of warmth and total relaxation, with the release of all muscle tension, invariably leads into a deep sleep if you are in a comfortable situation and allow yourself to drift off.

For most men, the resolution phase is also associated with a refractory period, during which the man is unable to become sexually aroused. This may last only a few minutes, or as long as hours, even days. Once a man is over the age of 50, he may only be able to ejaculate once in 24 hours.

Variation in sexual response

A variety of factors, including mood, surroundings and feelings for the partner, can influence the intensity of response at a particular moment. There can also be a wide variation in the timing of the excitation and plateau phases between different individuals and in one man on different occasions.

In addition, ejaculation may not always be the most pleasurable moment. Powerful reflex pelvic muscle contractions occurring either before or after ejaculation can be more satisfying, with ejaculation itself coming as rather an anti-climax!

Dr Bernard Zilbergeld, in his book *Men and Sex*, emphasises that an orgasmic experience can be heightened by learning to relax more during sex, by focusing on bodily sensations and by avoiding the tendency to restrict movements, breathing and noise. Spending more time stimulating your partner during your plateau phase can also enhance your orgasm.

It is important to disregard the popular myth that having reached the plateau phase, you are obliged to go on to orgasm. Although stopping love-making or masturbation at this stage may occasionally cause soreness or discomfort in the testicles, this is not in any way harmful.

Conception in women

Conception begins with the fertilisation of an ovum (egg) by one of the thousands of sperm that have survived the journey up the woman's vagina, through the cervix and uterus (womb) and into a fallopian tube. The fertilised ovum then has to implant itself successfully within the lining of the uterus for conception to be complete and an embryo to develop into a baby.

Passage of the egg

Around the middle of a woman's menstrual cycle, 14 days before the start of her next menstrual period, an egg is released from one or other ovary. Following ovulation, the egg is drawn into the nearby open end of the fallopian tube to begin its journey towards the uterus.

Rhythmic contractions of the muscles in the fallopian tube wall propel the egg along. It takes about four days for the egg to reach the cavity of the uterus. If it is not fertilised, it breaks up and is lost with the next menstrual period.

Passage of the sperm

Within 30 seconds of ejaculation during unprotected sexual intercourse, several million of the 100 million sperm released will have reached the uterus. Their passage through the cervix is assisted by a combination of the force of ejaculation, reflex contractions of the female pelvic muscles and, most importantly, the powerful swimming motion of the sperm tails.

Those sperm unable to penetrate the mucus barrier across the cervix remain in the vagina and soon die off. In fact, for much of a woman's menstrual cycle, apart from a few days around ovulation, this barrier is of a consistency that usually keeps out all the sperm anyway.

Of the few thousand sperm which survive the swim up the uterus cavity, only a few hundred reach the fallopian tube and have the chance to achieve fertilisation.

Fertilisation

Usually, just one sperm fuses with the egg. As the head of the sperm strikes the outer surface of the egg, a thin cap overlying the sperm's genetic material bursts to release enzymes which assist its penetration of the substance surrounding the ovum's genetic material.

Once the sperm head is fixed, the rest of the sperm becomes detached and, following fusion of the two collections of genetic material, the resulting zygote develops a protective covering to prevent other sperm from penetrating.

The possibility of fertilisation depends on timing, with the egg surviving in the upper part of the fallopian tube for a maximum of only 24 hours and sperm surviving for a maximum of seven days inside one of the fallopian tubes. To implant successfully, the zygote normally has to develop for another day or two, through a series of cell divisions, which is why conception is more likely if fertilisation occurs well up the fallopian tube and not too close to the uterus.

However, owing to variations in the time of ovulation and how long the egg and sperm can actually survive, the fertile period may be as long as ten days of the menstrual cycle.

Growing up

The most rapid phase of human body growth and development occurs inside the uterus, from the moment of conception onwards. Initially, body cells proliferate dramatically through a continuous process of cell division, with cell numbers doubling each time the cells divide. Then, as a result of the genetic blueprint in each cell, different body parts and organs begin to take shape. By the end of the first three months of pregnancy, the foetus is recognisable as a tiny human being and all the major organs will have formed. Over the remaining six months the baby grows steadily in size.

Infancy is also a period of rapid body growth, with the baby usually tripling in birth weight over the first year. Height generally increases at a steady rate of 5–8 cm each year after the age of two. In addition to growing taller and heavier, children go through a major change in body proportions, with their trunk and limbs catching up in relation to the size of their head.

Although all the various body organs are present at birth, many of them are immature in terms of both their structure and their function. An important part of early growth and development is therefore a steady maturation of these different organs. For example, most of the brain has grown before birth, but considerable changes in its internal structure, as well as in the rest of the nervous system, are necessary for the development of essential skills. Much of this maturation process involves the formation of new connections between nerves and is dependent on the brain receiving adequate and reliable stimulation through all five senses – touch, smell, taste, sight and hearing.

CONTROL OF GROWTH AND DEVELOPMENT

Both the external and internal body changes that occur as a normal part of growth and development depend primarily on the action of growth hormone, which is produced by the pituitary gland at the base of the brain. Growth hormone stimulates the formation of new protein in most body tissues, speeding up the process of cell proliferation to cause a steady increase in the bulk and complexity of these different structures. Interestingly, the influence of growth hormone on all cell changes appears to be most marked during sleep.

Changes at puberty

Male puberty is defined as the period of development during which a boy achieves physical sexual maturity and the ability to father children. In contrast, 'adolescence' includes the emotional as well as the physical changes that occur during the transition from boy to man. The start of puberty occurs when the pituitary gland at the base of the brain is stimulated to secrete gonadotrophin hormones. The gonadotrophins step up the production of testosterone by the testicles and within two years the boy will begin to notice the characteristic physical changes of puberty.

Puberty may start at any age from ten years old, but usually the onset is between 12 and 14, taking on average two-and-a-half years to complete. Boys who mature later or at a slower rate are understandably likely to be sensitive or worried about this. However, later maturity has no significance with regard to future virility or fertility.

Some of the changes of puberty generally occur in a predictable sequence, with an increase in the size of the testicles and scrotum being followed by enlargement of the penis. Pubic hair generally appears before armpit hair, with facial hair emerging later.

'WET DREAMS'

Waking up to find a damp, sticky patch of semen on the sheets can be a highly embarrassing experience for a teenage boy. However, this phenomenon of spontaneously ejaculating during the night is perfectly normal and unrelated to any previous sexual experience. Often the boy will be unable to remember actually having an erotic dream.

Spontaneous nocturnal emissions – or 'wet dreams', as they are more popularly known – begin at puberty. They may occur frequently until the boy finds some other regular sexual outlet, either masturbation or intercourse.

The majority of boys have reached about 80 per cent of their adult height before puberty. Nevertheless, there will usually be a noticeable pubertal growth spurt, along with all the other changes at puberty, which include:

- hair growth on the chest and abdomen
- muscle development, particularly around the upper chest and thighs
- voice breaks (drops to a lower pitch), due to enlargement of the larynx
- sperm production starts in the testicles.

Middle age

After childhood and puberty, the adult years appear to be a period in which nothing much goes on inside the body. However, constant activity occurs in body tissues throughout adult life, for example:

- the bones are living tissues that constantly renew their internal structure to remain strong and healthy
- muscle cells grow in size and develop more energy-producing units (mitochondria) if exercised regularly
- skin, intestinal lining and blood cells are continuously replaced
- intellectual powers may not peak until a man is in his 30s, or even older.

Growing old

The ageing process, during which body tissues and organs simply wear out, even if they have remained free of disease, normally starts to affect physical and intellectual capacity at some time after the age of 60 and progresses much faster in some men than in others. Ageing remains a mystery to doctors and scientists, although there are several theories as to the exact biological mechanisms involved, for example:

- a progressive decline in the body's immune system means that it is no longer able to defend itself as efficiently against bacteria, viruses and the growth of cancer cells
- a gradual build-up of toxins takes place inside the body
- the DNA templates, which control the copying of individual cells, are worn out, causing mistakes to occur in tissue and organ regeneration.

A number of changes may occur in the body as a normal part of ageing (see opposite). These changes are thought to be controlled, at least partly, by the genes you have inherited from your parents. However, a variety of lifestyle factors, such as cigarette-smoking, poor diet, lack of exercise, excessive alcohol consumption and regular exposure to strong sunlight, are known to accelerate the age-related degeneration of body organs and tissues.

Most men can slow down this natural decline by having a healthy lifestyle and remaining physically and intellectually active. Regular physical exercise can help to keep the heart, lungs, bones, muscles and circulation in good condition. Mental agility can often be preserved by ensuring that the brain is regularly stimulated with new ideas and activities.

It is certainly a mistake to regard illness, loss of mobility, loss of independence or the onset of dementia as an inevitable result of growing old; any persistent symptom of ill health should be reported to the doctor.

Ageing process

As you grow older, you may notice a variety of changes in your body and its performance, including:

- loss of muscle strength, bulk and endurance (stamina)
- increased joint stiffness
- injuries and wounds taking longer to heal
- reduced bone density, with increased risk of fracture
- compression of spinal bones and discs, causing loss of height
- wrinkling of skin, due to collagen degeneration
- increased likelihood of bruising, due to weakened skin capillaries
- impaired lung efficiency, resulting from reduced elasticity
- greying of hair as pigment-producing cells die off
- less efficient processing of alcohol and medication by the liver
- need for reading glasses, due to stiffness in eye lenses
- deafness to high-pitched sounds
- difficulties with short-term memory.

Sexual function in older men

While some older men prefer to cease their love-making, many others want to continue demonstrating love and affection for their partner in a physical way. Unfortunately, many older couples wrongly believe that an active sex life should end at 60 and they feel guilty or ashamed that what they are doing is in some way dirty.

In fact, assuming both partners want to make love, the enjoyment can actually improve in later life once the pressures of work and the worry of unwanted pregnancy have been left behind.

If an older man is having sexual problems, whether physical or psychological, he should start by consulting his doctor. For many of the common difficulties a solution can be found. For example, a change in medication, if relevant, may help improve potency (see pages 151–8).

Advice on love-making positions that are less physically stressful can overcome limitations caused by third-age health problems, such as osteoarthritis or angina. Referral to a professional counsellor (see pages 109–10) has helped many older couples to resolve their sexual fears and anxieties.

Chapter 2

How to stay physically healthy

MANY different factors determine whether you will remain physically healthy throughout your life. Some of the influences are clearly beyond your control, such as the genes you have inherited from your parents, the food you were given as a child, exposure to infection and whether you received all the recommended immunisations. However, many aspects of the way you live also affect your physical condition.

By adopting a healthy lifestyle, being aware of specific risks to your physical health and alert to the possible early-warning symptoms of illness, you will not only reduce your chances of dying young, you should also be able to enjoy a better quality of life well into old age.

Decisions you make about your diet, how much exercise you take and habits such as smoking and drinking alcohol can all directly harm or benefit your long-term physical health. You also need to know which symptoms to report to your doctor, how to keep an eye out for early-warning signs of disease through regular self-examination of different parts of your body and also when you should have the various screening tests designed to detect hidden diseases. Immunisation and accident prevention are also vitally important.

Diet and nutrition

A healthy diet

We need food to provide the energy that keeps our body cells alive and active. We also need food to supply the raw materials used for the growth, maintenance and repair of all the body's tissues and organs. However, eating is also an important part of our social lives and should therefore be a source of pleasure, not anxiety.

Unfortunately, since we became aware that diet can influence health, we have been bombarded with stories about the nutritional qualities of different products, most of these resulting from the food industry's desire to sell particular brands.

Healthy eating does not mean giving up all your favourite meals, nor spending hours obsessively studying the nutrient and calorie content of hundreds of different foods. The key to a healthy diet is simply variation and balance, with the emphasis on extending rather than restricting the range of foods you normally eat.

Variation and balance

To satisfy all your nutritional requirements by consuming the recommended intake of each vitamin and mineral and the correct mixture of carbohydrates, fats and proteins (see Glossary), you should try to eat as wide a variety of foods as possible. The easiest way to do this is to choose a range of foods each day from each of the five major food groups:

- breads, cereals and other grain products, such as rice
- fruits
- vegetables
- dairy produce, such as milk, cheese and yogurt
- plant proteins, such as dried beans, peas, nuts and seeds, and/or animal protein from eggs, fish, poultry or meat.

As well as having a balanced diet, healthy eating also means not taking in too much of any one kind of food and avoiding a surplus of calories, which will cause an increase in body weight. The ideal diet supplies sufficient calories to fulfil the body's energy requirements, which obviously depends on how much energy is being burned up through physical activity that day (see page 68). To achieve a healthy supply of both calories and nutrients, the recommended proportions of energy provided by carbohydrates, fats and proteins are 50–55 per cent, less than 30 per cent and about 15 per cent respectively.

Many men consume much more fat than this recommended intake. Also, most of the carbohydrate foods they eat contain predominantly refined sugars that tend to be high in calories, but low in fibre, vitamins and minerals. A high intake of fats, particularly saturated fats, raises blood cholesterol and increases the risk of heart disease. Too much fat, too many refined carbohydrates and too much alcohol (particularly beer or lager) are the reasons why so many men in the UK are overweight. Heavy consumption of sugar also encourages tooth decay.

Not eating enough fibre or drinking insufficient water can interfere with the efficiency of the digestive system, causing, for example, constipation and other bowel disorders.

To achieve a balanced diet, in addition to eating a wide variety of foods, you should therefore increase your fibre intake, cut down on fat and eat fewer sugary foods.

More fibre

A high intake of fibre is essential, not only to prevent constipation but also to help control the absorption of glucose (sugar) and digested fats from the intestine into the circulation. People who eat sufficient fibre are less likely to develop an abnormally high blood cholesterol level and less likely to suffer sudden changes in their blood sugar level, which can cause a variety of unpleasant symptoms such as headaches, dizziness and fatigue.

High-fibre foods fill you up without adding a lot of calories to your diet. Foods rich in fibre include wholegrain bread and cereal, fresh fruits and vegetables, brown rice and dried beans.

Less sugar

Foods packed with refined sugars, such as cakes, biscuits and jam, provide calories but are lacking in essential nutrients. In excess, they increase the risk of obesity and tooth decay. It is important to remember that many canned products, including certain brands of soup, baked beans, vegetables and fruits, contain a lot of added sugar, as does ketchup, because sugar is often used as a food preservative.

Easy ways to cut down your sugar intake are to pick unsweetened or artificially sweetened products, drink low-calorie soft drinks or water and avoid adding sugar to tea or coffee.

Less fat

Having some fat in the diet is essential as a source of vitamins A, D, E and K and to provide chemicals used in the production of new cells and hormones. However, to reduce the risk of obesity and heart disease, no more than 30 per cent of your energy intake should come from fat. Also, when you are eating or cooking with fat, try to choose mainly unsaturated rather than saturated fats whenever possible.

Saturated fat, which is found in meat, milk, cheese and butter and which is added to many processed foods, is converted in the liver to cholesterol. A build-up of cholesterol results in the walls of the arteries furring up with deposits of fat. Unsaturated fats, found in oily fish, nuts, margarine and most types of vegetable oil, do not increase cholesterol production and are thought to have a protective effect on the heart and blood vessels.

To keep your saturated fat intake down:

- eat lean meats such as chicken (without the skin), fish, liver and kidney
- limit your consumption of processed meats
- trim off the visible fat before cooking meat
- bulk out red meat dishes with a vegetable protein, such as red kidney beans
- cut down on fried food, and always use a polyunsaturated vegetable oil when you do fry
- use low-fat spreads and cheeses
- drink semi-skimmed rather than whole milk
- eat a maximum of four eggs each week – they are rich in cholesterol
- when you eat out, remember that sauces, gravies and dressings are usually full of fat
- avoid puddings and pastries, which are also loaded with fat.

Less salt

Most people eat far more salt than they need. In some individuals this may be a factor in the development of abnormally high blood pressure. Anyone with high blood pressure or heart failure is usually advised to cut down their salt intake because it can make both these disorders worse.

To limit the amount of salty foods you eat:

- avoid processed foods which contain a lot of salt, such as certain canned vegetables, soups and ketchups
- don't add salt (or add less) to your cooking and don't put salt on your food at the table
- beware pickles, chutneys, sausages, bacon, beefburgers, and some cheeses and butters which have a high salt content
- use a salt substitute – but not in excess.

Healthy eating habits

It is not just what you eat but also the way you eat your food that can influence your health. Eating virtually nothing during the day and then a large meal late in the evening, for example, is a common reason for putting on weight. Your body's metabolism works more efficiently on a regular supply of food energy. Starving yourself just causes the chemical activities in the cells that burn up calories to switch off. Also, you should take time out to rest and relax during and for at least half an hour after a meal and avoid vigorous exercise for up to three hours. Otherwise, you are likely to end up with indigestion, heartburn or wind.

Choosing a healthy snack

Unfortunately, a lot of the popular convenience foods, which are either ready to eat or quick and easy to prepare, do not meet the requirements for a healthy diet. They tend to be high in calories and contain a lot of saturated fat plus added sugar or salt; they are also usually low in fibre and short on essential nutrients. While the occasional unhealthy snack will not do any harm, eaten regularly this type of food increases your chance of becoming overweight and deficient in certain vitamins and minerals.

Many healthy and nutritious convenience foods are now available. It is a good idea before buying, therefore, to check the label for the fat, sugar and salt content. Also, remember that glucose, fructose, maltose and caramel are just different sorts of sugar.

Rather than snacking on crisps, cakes, biscuits and sweets, it is better to chew on a piece of fresh fruit or a raw vegetable like a carrot. If you make a sandwich, use wholegrain bread and a low-fat spread, then choose a lean filling such as low-fat cottage cheese or tuna.

Fast foods, like most convenience foods, also tend to be high in calories, saturated fat and salt, and low in fibre. Although they do provide many essential nutrients, including protein, some vitamins and minerals, fast foods are often lacking in vitamin A, vitamin C and calcium. When ordering fast food, watch out for the high-fat, calorie-rich sauces that often accompany a burger. And, even though chicken and fish are leaner meats than beef, when they are served as fast food they are generally fried in fat-rich batter. To balance the meal, have a side-salad without dressing and choose water rather than a regular soft drink.

Nutritional needs throughout life

A range of nutrients which must be present in the diet to maintain good health has been identified. For most of these vitamins and minerals, a recommended daily intake has been calculated, which represents the average quantity of that nutrient which each person should consume every day. This should satisfy the nutritional needs of around 97 per cent of the population without overdosing those who actually require less.

Table 1

Reference Nutrient Intakes (RNIs) – daily recommended consumption for adult males (19–50 years)

Vitamin A	0.7mg
Thiamine	1.0mg
Riboflavin	1.3mg
Niacin	17mg
Pantothenic acid	No recommendation – deficiency unknown
Vitamin B_6	1.4mg
Vitamin B_{12}	1.5mcg
Biotin	No RNI (suggested daily intake 10–200mcg)
Folic acid	200mcg
Vitamin C	40mg
Vitamin D	No RNI between 4 and 65 years
Vitamin E	No recommendation (suggested daily intake of alpha-tocopherol 3–4mg)
Vitamin K	1mcg per kg body weight
Calcium	700mg
Iodine	140mcg
Iron	8.7mg
Magnesium	300mg
Potassium	3.5g
Selenium	75mcg
Zinc	9.5mg
Phosphorus	550mg
Sodium	1.6g
Chloride	2.5g
Copper	1.2mg

These figures, known as Reference Nutrient Intakes (RNIs), which have replaced the old units of nutritional value, Recommended Daily Amounts (RDAs), are tabulated above for adult males aged between 19 and 50 years. Each RNI is a recommendation for the whole of this group of men, but it will not be exactly correct for all of them. This is because other factors, such as lifestyle and the state of a person's health, also influence nutrient requirements. However, if your intake of a nutrient is well below its RNI, there is certainly a risk of developing symptoms of deficiency.

To reduce the risk of illness as you get older and to boost your recovery after an illness, it is essential to continue to eat a healthy diet. It may also be necessary to adapt your eating habits to compensate for changes in your body that occur as a normal part of the ageing process.

TABLE 2: Common nutrient deficiencies in elderly men

Nutrient	Cause of deficiency (in addition to low intake)	Food source
Iron	Reduced absorption from ageing digestive system	Wholegrain cereals, green leafy vegetables, liver, fish and meat
Thiamine	Ageing increases requirement	Wholegrain bread and cereals, brown rice, beans, nuts, fish and liver
Calcium	Reduced absorption from ageing digestive system	Green leafy vegetables, dairy produce, eggs and fish with edible bones
Vitamin D	Lack of sunlight if housebound	Eggs, margarine and oily fish (sardines, tuna and herring)
Vitamin C	Lack of and overcooking vegetables and fruit	Fresh vegetables and fruit (particularly citrus)

Although older men usually continue to eat a sufficient amount of food, their diet is typically lacking in variety and balance, particularly for those men living alone who cook for themselves. They often start to rely on processed or convenience foods, which are a lot easier to buy and prepare, but may cost more than fresh products.

Some of the more common nutrient deficiencies found in elderly men are listed above, with advice on which foods should be eaten to prevent or correct each of these deficiencies.

Calorie requirements in men

Your body needs a certain amount of energy from food (measured in calories) to maintain vital physical and chemical functions both at rest and during exercise, to keep itself warm and also to build and repair different tissues, such as bone and muscle. For most healthy men, average daily calorie requirements are calculated from age and general level of physical activity (see Table A). The number of calories burned up per hour by the average man taking part in a variety of different activities has also been measured (see Table B). With this information, you should be able to work out roughly the calories you need to suit your particular requirements.

TABLE A: Average calorie requirements for men

Age	Lifestyle	Calories/day
18–35 years	Inactive	2,500
	Active	3,000
	Very active	3,500
36–70 years	Inactive	2,400
	Active	2,900
	Very active	3,400
70+ years	Inactive	2,200
	Active	2,500

Note These are average values; there are a few people who have a slow metabolism and therefore require less food energy to keep their body running. Also, there are a few 'fast burners' who do not put on weight even though eating large amounts of calories.

Men who consistently consume more calories than they need for their daily physical activity and body maintenance requirements will inevitably put on weight. Surplus food is converted into fat, which is then deposited around the body, particularly the abdomen, where it forms the familiar paunch.

Calorie needs in older men

As the body ages, its energy requirements decrease. One reason is the tendency to take less vigorous exercise in later life. In addition, a pro-

TABLE B: Calorie consumption per hour of activity

Activity	Calories burned
Sleeping	65
Writing	100
Walking	250
Brisk walking	300
Cycling	300
Slow running	400
Swimming	500
Squash	650
Fast running	650

Note Some of these values clearly depend on the amount of effort put in, for example, swimming would burn 500 calories/hour only if you were doing continuous lengths of the pool.

gressive reduction in the basal metabolic rate (the energy used up by the body to maintain vital functions, such as breathing and heartbeat) occurs as a normal part of the ageing process. This explains why older men may put on weight unless they adjust their eating and exercise habits.

Nutrient supplements

Most men obtain the recommended amounts (see page 66) of vitamins and minerals simply by eating a varied and balanced diet. If you eat the sort of healthy diet described earlier, taking a supplement is unlikely to make any significant difference to your health.

However, anyone who eats a lot of processed or highly refined foods runs the risk of becoming marginally deficient in a variety of nutrients, including vitamins B_6 and E, chromium, zinc, copper and selenium. A lot of vague symptoms and minor skin problems are thought to be due to a marginal deficiency in one or more nutrients, but this can only be confirmed by a doctor arranging specific blood tests.

A variety of other conditions or situations can also lead to vitamin or mineral deficiency:

- elderly men often neglect their diet for the reasons described earlier
- men struggling with poverty, alcoholism, drug abuse and mental illness are all likely to have an inadequate diet

- chronic diseases of the stomach, intestine, pancreas or liver may interfere with either the absorption or digestion of a particular nutrient; kidney failure can lead to a deficiency of potassium, magnesium, calcium and vitamin D
- long-term medication may upset the absorption or metabolism of a specific nutrient: for example, some anti-epilepsy drugs increase the need for folic acid and vitamin D
- a drastic weight-reducing diet, in which there is a low intake of food or limitations on the types of food being eaten, can be inadequate nutritionally.

How to choose a supplement

It is best to consult your doctor before starting to take any nutrient supplement. Products which contain only one type of vitamin or mineral may cause problems by increasing the body's demand for other nutrients. Multi-vitamin and mineral preparations contain a variety of nutrients in different doses and combinations, which can be confusing.

Some brands of supplement contain several times the recommended daily dose of a nutrient, which in certain circumstances could lead to unpleasant adverse effects. Too much of a vitamin or mineral can do more harm than good. For example, in large amounts:

- vitamin B_6 (pyridoxine) may damage nerves, causing numbness, pins and needles and weakness
- vitamin D may cause nausea, vomiting and muscle spasm
- vitamin A may result in skin irritation and hair loss
- iron may upset the digestive system, leading to diarrhoea or constipation.

An unhealthy diet cannot be made healthy by taking a nutrient supplement. The right mixture of foods in a balanced diet provides not only the required vitamins and minerals, but also the correct proportion of fat, protein, carbohydrate and fibre.

Losing weight

An accurate way to assess whether you are carrying too much weight is to calculate your Body Mass Index (BMI). This figure is derived by dividing your weight, measured in kilograms, by the square of your height, measured in metres (BMI = W/H^2). For example, a man who weighs 83kg and is 1.83m tall would have a BMI of 24.78 (i.e. 83 ÷ [1.83 x 1.83]).

If your BMI is between 20 and 25, this is considered healthy. However, a BMI between 25 and 30 is a sign of being overweight, and over 30 is defined as obese. At least 30 per cent of men in the UK are overweight and almost 5 per cent are in the obese category.

Overweight men tend to have less energy, they are more likely to become overheated and breathless during exercise, their ankles are more likely to swell and the joints in their back and legs are more likely to ache. Overweight and obese men are more vulnerable to:

- high blood pressure
- high blood cholesterol
- gallstones
- varicose veins
- osteoarthritis
- coronary heart disease
- diabetes
- stroke.

Weight-reducing diets

Most men who are overweight are not suffering from any hormonal or metabolic disorder, they simply have a calorie intake that consistently exceeds their energy requirements. This is usually due to a combination of over-eating and not taking enough exercise to burn off the excess calories.

Tackling the problem of over-eating is as difficult for most men as giving up smoking or cutting down on alcohol. The fact that no single diet is universally successful is reflected by the large numbers of popular diet books on sale, each recommending different types of diet. However, basic principles of successful weight reduction are:

- first set yourself a realistic target weight and aim to lose about one kilogram each week
- consider joining a slimming group to help keep you motivated
- choose a varied, balanced diet (as described earlier) – the sort of diet that you can follow as a normal part of your life
- eat two to three proper small meals, don't miss out a meal and don't snack in between; if you must snack, choose healthy foods

- increase your intake of fibre-rich, starchy foods, such as potatoes, rice and pasta (with a tomato-based rather than creamy sauce)
- cut down on refined, sugary foods
- eat less fat, particularly saturated fat
- cut down on alcohol (particularly beer and lager), switch to low-calorie soft drinks and drink plenty of water
- eat slowly and cut up your food into small pieces so that it takes longer to eat; use a smaller plate
- don't eat while you are reading or watching TV.

When you achieve your target weight, it is important not to slip back into your previous unhealthy eating habits. Unfortunately, many men often end up weighing more than they did before they originally started to diet. This cycle of weight loss followed by weight gain is now thought to be more damaging to physical health than remaining consistently overweight.

EXERCISE

Losing weight is not just about diet and healthy nutrition: regular strenuous exercise is also important. Brisk walking, swimming and cycling are all good activities to burn up extra calories and reduce your body's fat stores. Regular physical activity also raises your basal metabolic rate (see Glossary), so that you burn up more calories at rest. Also, a vigorous workout can depress appetite and take your mind off the urge to snack.

Warning Consult your doctor before beginning any exercise programme if you are overweight.

Drugs to help weight reduction

Trying to eat healthier foods and avoid over-eating is not easy, which is why some men ask their doctor for a drug to help them lose weight. Up until September 1998, two main types of slimming tablet were available on prescription: a bulking agent (methylcellulose), which taken with water before a meal swells inside the stomach to make you feel full and therefore less hungry, and stimulants which suppress appetite by acting on the hypothalamus at the base of the brain.

Because of worries about side-effects on the heart, the only stimulant currently available on prescription is phentermine.

However, a new anti-obesity drug – a lipase inhibitor known as orlistat (Xenical) – promotes weight loss and prevents weight regain by reducing the absorption of fat from food as it passes through the digestive system. Like other slimming drugs, orlistat has to be taken in conjunction with a calorie-controlled diet.

Sports nutrition

It is a common misconception that if you play a lot of sport or train hard you need to take some form of nutrient supplement. Although it is true that the more active a man is, the higher his calorie intake should be, just eating a varied balanced diet should satisfy the body's demand for all the different vitamins, minerals, amino acids and other nutrients. Taking a supplement will not normally make any difference to physical fitness, nor to the speed of recovery after intense training or an injury.

Try to eat at least three hours before you exercise. If you eat less than an hour before, you are likely to feel nauseous and uncomfortable because food is still in your stomach. If you haven't eaten for more than five hours, there is a good chance you could develop abdominal discomfort or feel light-headed.

The best type of food to eat if you plan to exercise later is starchy carbohydrate, such as pasta or potatoes. In contrast with fat- and protein-rich foods, such as steak, carbohydrates are digested and absorbed quickly to provide an immediate supply of energy for the muscle cells in the form of glucose (sugar).

Drink enough fluids
Body water is lost when you perspire during strenuous exercise. It is therefore important to drink enough fluids before and after exercise to avoid becoming dehydrated. In hot and humid conditions, or if you are involved in an activity that lasts longer than 45 minutes, it is a good idea to drink small amounts of liquid at regular intervals throughout the exercise.

Feeling thirsty is not a reliable guide to how much fluid you need, so get into the habit of drinking liquids as a normal part of your exercise routine. A good example of fluid replacement being taken seriously is the professional tennis player who drinks something on virtually every changeover. Water is the best drink to prevent dehydration during exercise. Have one or two glasses about half an hour before you start to make sure your tissues begin with a good supply of fluid. If you break off for a rest period after 30–45 minutes, drink another glass. For a continuous activity lasting longer than one hour, such as running a marathon or playing tennis, drink at regular intervals but take only small amounts.

These precautions should prevent the onset of dehydration, which might otherwise spoil both your enjoyment and your performance. Once the exercise is over, drink yet more water, particularly if you have been perspiring heavily.

A high-energy sports drink containing sugar may help keep your muscles supplied with glucose during an endurance event lasting two hours or more, such as running a marathon. However, it is not needed for most sporting activities and there is no scientific evidence to prove that a sports drink actually boosts performance.

A Food Commission report expressed concern at the large amounts of added sugar in sports drinks. One serving of some of the more popular brands provides the equivalent of between eight and 24 lumps of sugar, which is certainly not part of a healthy diet – however many calories you intend to burn up. It is also possible that this high sugar content could encourage dehydration by drawing water out of the bloodstream into the stomach to dilute the drink.

Coffee, tea and cola drinks, containing caffeine, are best avoided because caffeine acts as a diuretic, which removes more body water in the urine. Although caffeine in high doses is believed to have a stimulant effect on exercise performance, you would need to take it as a concentrated tablet to achieve any benefit, and such a large amount is regarded as a prohibited drug in most sports. Remember also that alcohol is a diuretic, which diverts more body water into the urine, increasing the chance of dehydration. You should therefore delay drinking alcohol after exercise until you have restored your body fluids with water.

Salt tablets

Salt replacement is needed only if you are taking part in a long strenuous activity in a hot or humid environment and you are having to drink large amounts of fluid to stay hydrated. Under normal circumstances your body is able to compensate for the salt lost in sweat simply by reducing the amount of salt passed out in the urine.

There is a tendency to blame cramp on lack of salt, but the real reason is more likely to be muscle fatigue or injury. In fact, taking salt tablets when you don't need them may actually bring on an attack of cramp.

Exercise and keeping fit

First, it is important not to confuse good health with good fitness. Rarely being ill does not automatically imply that you are in good physical condition. Likewise, being physically fit is not the same as sporting excellence – you do not have to train for hours in order to improve and maintain your fitness. Rather than visiting a gym or buying special equipment, one easy way to increase the amount of exercise you take is to walk or cycle part of the way to work.

A basic definition of fitness is the ability to cope easily with the physical workload of normal daily activities, without becoming unduly breathless or exhausted, and still have extra energy in reserve to meet any sudden unexpected demand: for example, to be able to carry heavy bags and run for the bus. Your general level of fitness is determined by the efficiency of your heart, lungs, circulation and muscles, which in turn is influenced by how regularly you exercise in a sustained and vigorous way.

Starting a fitness programme

Before starting any strenuous physical activity to get fit, it is advisable to have a check-up from your doctor first if:

- you are over 35 and have done very little exercise for a few years
- you are over 60 years old
- you are significantly overweight
- you are a smoker
- someone in your immediate family developed heart disease before the age of 40
- you are under medical treatment or supervision for high blood pressure, a heart condition, diabetes or any other long-term disease.

These precautions allow your doctor to detect any disorder that could make over-exerting yourself dangerous and to advise which exercises are suitable in your particular circumstances.

Having made the decision to start and been given the go-ahead by your doctor (if necessary), you then need to devise your own fitness programme. Ideally, this should include a mixture of exercises designed to improve all three components of your fitness: endurance, strength and flexibility.

When you first begin exercising, do not try to push yourself too hard too soon. Your routine should make you a little breathless, but not gasping for air; tired, but not completely exhausted. Slowly, over a period of several weeks, increase the amount of time and effort you put in as your level of fitness improves.

Strength

Strength is the ability to use muscle force to lift, carry, push or pull a heavy load. Your body contains over 600 muscles to enable it to perform hundreds of different movements. Depending on your build, this muscle tissue may represent anything between one-quarter and one-half of your body weight. If your muscles are weak and out of condition, any activity for which strength is important will be more difficult to perform.

An easy way to assess your muscle strength is to count how many sit-ups you can perform in one minute. It is important to keep your knees bent to avoid straining your lower back and your hands against the side of your head, not behind as this can strain the neck. Around 20–25 sit-ups is average for men under the age of 50; much less than this and you need to strengthen your abdominal muscles.

Flexibility

Flexibility is the ability to stretch, bend or twist through a wide range of movements. This is determined by the degree of suppleness of your joints and the elasticity of your muscles and tendons. A lack of flexibility increases the risk of a sprain or strain resulting from a sudden or violent movement. Tight back and leg muscles can lead to back pain and stiffness after exercise.

To measure your flexibility, try the following sit and reach test. Sitting on the floor with your legs slightly apart and keeping your back and knees straight, lean forward slowly from your waist. If you are unable to get close to touching your heels, you may benefit from stretching exercises to improve the flexibility of your back and hamstring muscles (see 'Flexibility exercises', pages 80–1).

Endurance

Endurance is the ability to keep on exercising without stopping to rest. Good endurance depends on the efficiency and performance of your heart, lungs, muscles and circulation. Anyone whose endurance is low will develop muscle fatigue and loss of co-ordination during prolonged exercise, increasing the risk of sustaining an injury.

To test your own endurance level, try walking briskly or jogging for about a mile or, alternatively, walk at a steady pace up three flights of stairs. If you have to stop during this activity to catch your breath, or because your legs are aching, or you end up too breathless to talk properly, you would benefit from exercises to enhance your endurance.

Checking the fitness of your heart

You can check the fitness of your heart by first counting your resting pulse and then measuring your pulse recovery 30 seconds after a session of strenuous exercise. To take your pulse, press your fingertips firmly against the artery on the front of your wrist at the base of your thumb. Count the number of beats over a 15-second period and multiply by four to calculate your heart rate per minute.

The most reliable reading of your resting pulse is the one taken when you have just woken up in the morning. In general, a fit heart is associated with a slow, strong and regular pulse. Men have a slightly higher resting pulse than women, and the values increase a little with age. The table below shows the approximate relationship for men between age, resting pulse and fitness level.

TABLE 3: Resting pulse rates in men

	Age	20–29	30–39	40–49	50+
Fitness level	Excellent	≤59	≤63	≤65	≤67
	Good	60–69	64–71	66–73	68–75
	Fair	70–85	72–85	74–89	76–89
	Poor	≥86	≥86	≥90	≥90

Note If your resting pulse is 100 beats/minute or more, see your doctor as soon as possible.

Step-ups are the easiest type of strenuous exercise to perform indoors. Using a stair or stool about 20cm high, step up and down off it moving one foot after the other. Continue the exercise for at least three minutes at a rate of around 24 step-ups per minute. Then, after

30 seconds' rest check your pulse at the wrist. This time count over a 10-second period only and multiply the figure by six to calculate your heart rate per minute; any longer would allow the pulse to recover further. The table below shows the approximate relationship for men between age, pulse recovery at 30 seconds and fitness level.

TABLE 4: Pulse recovery in men at 30 seconds

	Age	20–29	30–39	40–49	50+
Fitness	Excellent	74	78	80	82
level	Good	76–84	80–86	82–88	84–90
	Fair	86–100	88–100	90–104	92–104
	Poor	>102	>102	>106	>106

Warning Do not perform step-ups if your starting pulse is 100 or over and stop this exercise at once if you develop any symptoms of heart strain (see pages 81–2).

How to stay motivated

The benefits to your future health from keeping fit are soon lost if you do not continue to exercise regularly. Unfortunately, as many as half of the men who start themselves on an exercise programme drop out within six months. Here are a few tips to help you stay motivated:

- set yourself short-term as well as long-term fitness goals that are not beyond your capabilities
- write down what you hope to achieve, e.g. losing a few kilograms in weight or being able to run for the bus again
- find an exercise partner so you can encourage each other
- choose activities you enjoy and find convenient to do
- vary your routine to avoid becoming bored
- have regular exercise slots at the same time in your weekly schedule
- keep a record of the type and amount of exercise you have been doing so you can monitor your progress
- during a repetitive exercise, count backwards from your target number to zero.

Endurance exercises

To improve your endurance, you need to participate in aerobic activities regularly, i.e. any form of prolonged exercise that can be performed continuously for at least 12 minutes. During aerobic exercise, the heart and lungs work hard enough to maintain a sufficient supply of oxygen to the muscles, allowing the muscle cells to continue functioning normally for a long period. Aerobic activities include jogging, brisk walking, skipping, swimming, dancing and cycling. Regular aerobic exercise carried out for around 20 minutes at a time, three times a week, enhances endurance by boosting the efficiency of your heart, lungs, muscles and circulation.

Target heart rate

To gauge how hard you need to work during aerobic activities to achieve the maximum benefit, you should aim to raise your pulse as near as possible to your target heart rate. When you first start a fitness programme, you are likely to find it impossible to reach this target without breaking the guidelines on not pushing yourself too hard.

Your target heart rate is the sum of your resting pulse plus half the difference between your resting pulse and the theoretical maximum pulse for your age. This theoretical maximum pulse is calculated by subtracting your age from 220. For example, a man of 40 with a resting pulse of 80 has a theoretical maximum pulse of 220 minus 40 which equals 180. Fifty per cent of the difference between his resting pulse and theoretical maximum is 180 minus 80, divided by two, which equals 50. Added to the resting pulse, 80 plus 50, produces a target heart rate of 130 beats per minute. To see how near you are to your target, take your pulse after a few minutes of aerobic activity. Count over a 10-second period and then multiply by six, otherwise your heart will have time to start slowing down again.

Strength exercises

Muscle-strengthening exercises will improve your body shape and posture by increasing muscle tone. They will also make it easier to move heavy loads. There are various types of strength exercises, including:

Multiple repetitions using small weights to improve muscle strength and tone, without significantly increasing muscle bulk. Start with weights light enough for you to be able to perform at least eight repetitions. Once you can cope easily with 12 repetitions in one minute, move on to a slightly heavier weight. It is important to perform each movement correctly, holding the weight at the furthest point for a count of two and breathing out at the same time. Leave a five-minute gap between each set of repetitions working a particular muscle group and rotate through a circuit of other muscle groups in the meantime. Three complete circuits of these different exercises are recommended for each workout.

Lifting heavy weights is the way to build up muscle bulk, performing just a few repetitions for each group of muscles because the exercise will be anaerobic (short, sharp burst of vigorous muscle activity which results in a build-up of lactic acid because the cells need more oxygen than can be supplied). The increase in bulk is due to the formation of more contracting strands inside each muscle fibre, making the fibre thicker, but there is no change in the actual number of muscle fibres.

Isometric exercises contract the muscle fibres, but without changing the length of the muscle, so there is no visible movement in that part of the body. This can be done either by holding part of the body in a fixed position against the pull of gravity, or by using one group of muscles to resist an attempted movement in another. These static exercises which boost tone and strength are unsuitable for anyone who has had a heart condition or stroke because they tend to raise blood pressure.

To reduce the risk of injury, always warm up with gentle stretching and loosening-up movements before starting any muscle-strengthening exercises. While it is usual for strength exercises to cause some burning discomfort, stop at once if you notice a sharp pain which could signal injury. Strength exercises are best done in a properly equipped gym, supervised by an experienced instructor. Children under the age of 14 should not be lifting heavy weights as a growing skeleton is more vulnerable to injury.

Flexibility exercises

Exercises to maintain and improve flexibility will help posture, counteract the generalised aches and stiffness associated with a sedentary lifestyle and reduce the chance of injury if you have to make a sudden or extreme movement. A range of stretching exercises should be carried out before or after any vigorous physical activity as part of warming up and cooling down (see opposite). Stretching exercises are also important if you are doing a regular muscle-strengthening programme as this training tends to tighten and shorten the muscles.

When you stretch, never bounce or jerk the muscle and never force the movement to a point where it becomes painful. Stretch until you feel a pull and hold this position for a count of ten. The most important muscle stretches involve the calf muscles, the front and back of the thighs, the front of the hips, the lower part of the back and the muscles across the chest and shoulders.

Figure 9: Muscle-stretching exercise

Exercising safely

Anyone who exercises or plays sport regularly is bound to pick up the occasional minor injury. However, while some of these injuries may be due to external causes beyond your control, such as foul play, many could be prevented by taking certain precautions, for example:

- always use the protective equipment available for a specific sport
- replace exercise shoes that have become excessively worn, or which no longer fit properly
- warm up with a routine of stretching and loosening-up exercises for at least ten minutes before the activity – this makes the tissues more elastic and therefore less vulnerable to injury
- cool down with muscle stretches and by continuing to move around for a few minutes after the activity to remove lactic acid from the muscles and thereby reduce subsequent stiffness and soreness
- make sure that playing equipment, such as the handle on a racquet or the grip on an oar, is the correct size for you to reduce the chance of a repetitive strain injury
- avoid alcohol or any drug that might make you feel dizzy or drowsy: the resultant loss of co-ordination or delay in reaction time could lead to an injury
- iron out any problems in your technique by consulting a coach or a coaching manual; many injuries are due to basic errors in the way a movement is performed.

An injury that remains painful, tender, stiff or swollen needs further treatment; otherwise, there is a risk of either making the injury worse or developing a second injury by trying to protect the first. Finally, an essential part of exercising safely is to be aware of warning symptoms that suggest you are overworking or damaging part of your body. Pain, soreness or stiffness in your muscles before you start an activity suggests that you should be allowing yourself a longer recovery time between training or playing sessions. Pain, stiffness or swelling in your joints could be the result of excessive jarring because you are not wearing cushioned insoles inside your exercise shoes.

Danger signals that you might be overtaxing your heart during strenuous exercise include:

- chest pain or pain in the neck or arms
- palpitations or skipped heart beats
- nausea, dizziness, light-headedness or feeling faint
- severe breathlessness
- extreme fatigue.

Stop exercising at once if you suffer any of the above symptoms while you are exercising and have a check-up from your doctor before continuing with your fitness programme.

Exercise and illness

Although there are a few acute medical conditions for which exercise is not recommended, such as infection and anaemia, with most chronic illnesses it is important to remain as physically active as possible. Participating in some form of regular exercise will often help minimise the amount of disability resulting from a particular disorder, as well as reducing the risk of developing complications. Even with diseases for which exercise does not have any direct benefit, staying active is still important to prevent the steady deterioration in general health that occurs with a progressive loss of fitness. Continuing to exercise is also good for morale.

If you have a chronic disorder such as asthma, diabetes, high blood pressure or arthritis, it is essential to see your doctor for a check-up and to obtain advice on which activities you can safely take part in before starting a fitness programme.

Even men who are confined to bed or a wheelchair can benefit from a regular routine of stretching and loosening-up exercises.

WARNING – EXERCISE AND INFECTION

Do not be tempted to continue exercising when you have symptoms of an infection, such as a sore throat, fever, swollen glands or a mucus-producing cough. Not only will your performance be below par, but with some viral infections, strenuous exercise can result in a dangerous complication, like myocarditis (inflammation of the heart).

Sports injuries and their treatment

With an ever-increasing number of men participating in sport, going to the gym or jogging to get fit, it is not surprising that there is also an associated epidemic of sports injuries. Unfortunately, many of the men who suffer a sports injury do not get the right advice or the best treatment to assist their recovery when they go to their GP or to the hospital accident and emergency department for treatment.

If you have not broken a bone, you will usually be sent home and told to rest, but often with no guidance on first-aid measures, when to start exercising again or what sort of exercises to do as you recover. In many cases, the injury will heal with rest, although, without a proper rehabilitation programme, as soon as you return to your normal sporting activities, the injury is likely to come back.

Most sports injuries involve minor damage to the soft tissues – muscles, ligaments, tendons or the lining of a joint – caused by overstretching. After any soft tissue injury, you should always follow the 'RICE' first-aid routine for the initial 48 hours. RICE stands for:

- **REST** – avoid exercise and any unnecessary movement to allow healing to start and reduce further bleeding and swelling. For an arm or shoulder injury, you can rest it in a sling; crutches or a stick can be used to keep weight off an injured leg
- **ICE** – a bag of frozen vegetables (or ice cubes) wrapped in a wet cloth or flannel should be applied to the injury every few hours for 10 minutes at a time to relieve pain, and to reduce bleeding and swelling by narrowing damaged blood vessels. Wash in a tepid shower and avoid hot baths, as heat during the first 48 hours will have the opposite effect from ice: increasing blood flow to make the swelling and bruising worse
- **COMPRESSION** – an elasticated stocking or crepe bandage will also help to reduce bleeding and swelling. The bandage should extend well above and below the injury but not be so tight that it causes numbness, tingling, pain or blanching of the skin
- **ELEVATION** – keeping the injured area raised (above the heart when possible) will minimise bleeding and swelling and help drain away fluid caused by inflammation of the damaged tissues. An arm injury can be elevated in a sling; a leg injury should be supported sitting with the foot up on a stool, or lying flat with the foot on cushions or a pillow.

Making a full recovery

After 48 hours and once the pain and swelling have subsided, you can begin gentle exercises, as long as movement does not make the pain worse. Exercises must include gentle stretching to restore full mobility and flexibility. Otherwise, the scar tissue left behind, which tends to shorten the muscle or tendon involved, is liable to tear again.

You will also need to do strengthening exercises to build up the muscles again, exercises to restore balance and co-ordination (particularly important after an ankle injury), and aerobic activity, such as swimming or using an exercise machine, to rebuild your fitness.

As the injury continues to heal, the time and effort put into these exercises can be increased. Do not make the common mistake of resting until the injury is pain-free and then going straight back to your sport without rehabilitation.

If you suffer persistent pain, tenderness, stiffness or swelling, you will need to see a doctor or a physiotherapist with an interest in sports injuries. It may be that you need additional treatment, such as massage, manipulation, ultrasound, laser treatment, anti-inflammatory drugs, a corticosteroid injection, or even surgery to make a full recovery.

Only a few sports injury clinics offer free treatment on the NHS. If you go to a private clinic, it is important to first check the cost for each session of treatment; usually the initial consultation will be more expensive than the follow-up appointments. Make sure you are given advice on exercises to do yourself at home, not just treatment at the clinic.

For further information on sports injury clinics in your area, contact the National Sports Medicine Institute.★

Body care

Skin, nails and hair

One important part of staying physically healthy is to take good care of your skin, nails and hair. If you look good, you are also likely to feel good. Eating a balanced, varied diet, as described earlier, and drinking sufficient amounts of water during the day will help keep your skin, hair and nails in good condition. It is also important, however, not to neglect these parts of your body through inadequate personal care or other unhealthy habits.

Skin-care tips

- make sure your diet contains plenty of fresh fruit and vegetables
- drink at least eight glasses of non-carbonated water every day (caffeine-containing drinks, such as tea, coffee and cola, are not a substitute as they increase water loss in the urine)
- if you smoke, give up, as this encourages premature wrinkling
- wash regularly with a mild soap and water to remove dirt and dead skin
- rinse off all soap thoroughly

- do not spend too long in the bath or shower and make sure that the water is not too hot
- use a moisturiser each time you wash if you suffer from dry skin
- dry carefully between your fingers and toes
- cover up with tightly woven, cotton clothing when you are out in the sun; put a sunscreen with a high protection factor on any exposed skin; also, wear a wide-brimmed hat
- wrap up well in cold, windy weather
- avoid direct contact with irritant substances, such as household cleaners and cement, by wearing protective gloves.

Nail-care tips

- don't cut your nails too short
- cut your toenails straight across to stop them ingrowing
- soften your nails in warm water before cutting them
- to protect against nail infection, wear rubber gloves when your hands are being continually immersed in water
- see a doctor if your nails become discoloured or start to crumble as this could be due to a treatable fungal infection.

Hair-care tips

- shampoo your hair regularly to remove any build-up of dirt and grease
- massage your scalp to stimulate blood flow and relax tension
- rinse hair thoroughly under a shower stream if possible
- use a conditioner to smooth the outer surface of the hairs
- keep the hairdryer at least 15cm away to avoid heat damage
- leave your hair slightly damp
- don't brush your hair when it is wet, use a wide-toothed comb; hair is at its weakest when wet
- avoid over-vigorous rubbing of wet hair, which can cause split ends and tangling
- beware of using harsh anti-dandruff shampoos – ask your barber or hairdresser for advice on a suitable preparation.

Looking after your feet

Much of the advice on foot care relates to the prevention of athlete's foot, which is covered in detail in Chapter 6. In addition:

- use a pumice stone to remove dead skin from the heels and balls of your feet
- discard shoes that are worn beyond repair, or no longer fit properly
- wear natural materials, such as cotton socks and leather shoes, to reduce sweating. If you suffer from smelly feet, wear insoles made of activated charcoal, which absorb sweat and odour particles
- change socks daily to prevent foot odour – a powder containing an antibacterial drug to reduce the numbers of skin bacteria along with an antioxidant to slow down the chemical breakdown of sweat can also help
- if you develop a foot problem, such as a corn, callus or bunion, see a member of the Society of Chiropodists★ (who will have the qualification SRCh) or a member of the British Chiropody Association.★

Eye-care tips

It is important to have a routine eye test at least every two years, or sooner if you notice any change in your vision (see pages 223–5). Your sight is precious and irreplaceable, so take good care of your eyes:

- use eye protection if you work with dangerous chemicals or high-speed machinery
- have a light shining on to the page when you are reading or writing, preferably from behind one of your shoulders
- rest your eyes frequently during close work, particularly when using a VDU, by staring into space for a few seconds every 15 minutes to prevent eye strain
- when watching TV, sit at least five feet from the screen
- wear sunglasses in strong sunlight to cut down glare
- a tinted visor is essential when welding as the intense light can damage the eyes
- fit spectacles worn for sport with plastic lenses, otherwise switch to contact lenses
- wear protective goggles to play squash
- wear goggles to help prevent eye irritation if you are swimming in a highly chlorinated pool
- avoid rubbing your eyes as this is a common way of picking up infection

- ask your pharmacist to recommend eye drops or an eye bath for tired, dry or sore eyes, but if the discomfort persists have your eyes checked by an optician or doctor.

Taking care of teeth and gums

Clean, healthy teeth and gums will make you look good and feel more self-confident. In addition to regular visits to the dentist at least once or twice a year, you should:

- brush your teeth and gums two or three times a day after meals, using a fluoride toothpaste, to remove the debris between the teeth and gums where plaque forms
- use dental floss or tape and toothpicks with care to avoid damaging the gums
- consider using stimulator tips made of rubber to improve the circulation through the gums
- cut down on sugary foods
- eat cheese at the end of a meal to neutralise mouth acids
- ask your dentist about fluoride supplements.

D-i-y health checks

Regular self-examination of your testicles, skin and mouth is an essential part of helping yourself to stay physically healthy. You are the person most familiar with your body and its appearance, shape and feel and are therefore in the best position to notice the early-warning signs of diseases such as cancer.

Examining your testicles

All men should get into the habit of regularly examining their testicles for the appearance of lumps or irregularities, or a change in their size, shape or firmness, in the same way that women are encouraged to examine their breasts. Although cancer of the testicle is relatively rare compared with other types of cancer, it is still the most common cancer in young men aged between 20 and 35. If detected early, it is one of the easiest to cure.

Self-examination of the testicles is best performed after a warm bath or shower, when the scrotal skin is loose and relaxed. Support the scrotum and testicles in the palm of the hand to check their weight and size. Using both hands, gently roll each testicle in turn between the thumb and index and middle fingers. Any change in either testicle should be reported to your doctor as soon as possible.

Examining your skin

A regular skin check is important, not only to detect cancer but also to identify any change that might indicate some other health problem. As with testicular cancer, the sooner skin cancer is discovered and treated, the better the chance of achieving a complete cure.

Skin self-examination is particularly important for those men who have a greater risk of skin cancer, for example because they have:

- a fair complexion
- been regularly exposed to strong sunlight without covering up
- a large number of moles
- moles which are large, irregular in shape and patchy in colour
- a previous skin cancer
- a close relative who has had skin cancer.

Warning signs to look out for during a skin check include: a slowly growing lump or bump, a change in skin texture or colour, a mole or blemish that has changed in shape, size or colour, or that has started to itch or bleed, a sore or ulcer that has failed to heal within three weeks and the sudden appearance of a new mole.

Checking inside your mouth

In addition to regular appointments with your dentist, it is a good idea to examine the inside of your own mouth regularly using a mirror. This is particularly important for men who smoke or drink heavily, as they are more likely to develop a mouth cancer. Changes in the mouth to look out for and report to your dentist or doctor include:

- recurrent mouth or gum bleeding
- the appearance of a new lump or swelling
- a persistent white patch, which may be a pre-cancerous condition (leukoplakia)
- any sore area on the lip, gum or inside of the mouth that fails to heal within three weeks
- numbness or pain inside the mouth for no apparent reason.

Cancer warning symptoms

As many as one in three men will develop cancer at some time in their lives. It is therefore important to be alert to the various early-warning symptoms of cancer. The point is not to become a neurotic hypochondriac, totally obsessed with the idea that any vague symptom you might develop is almost certainly the result of cancer, but to know which specific symptoms to have checked out by your doctor.

The actual cause of one of these symptoms is often something much less serious. However, ruling out cancer will put your mind at rest and in those few cases where cancer is confirmed, treatment can be started before too much damage is done and before the cancer has advanced to a stage where it can no longer be dealt with successfully. Some cancer early-warning symptoms to be aware of are:

- coughing up blood
- hoarseness that recurs or persists for longer than one week
- unexplained lumps or bumps
- swallowing difficulty that persists
- abdominal pain that recurs or persists
- unexplained constipation or diarrhoea that is prolonged for more than one week
- rectal bleeding, particularly when blood is mixed with faeces
- blood in urine
- unexplained weight loss
- headaches that persist or recur
- change in shape, size or firmness of a testicle
- bruising without injury
- a mole that changes shape, size or colour, bleeds or itches
- a scab, sore or ulcer that fails to heal within three weeks
- a persistent white patch inside the mouth.

Routine check-ups

Eye tests

Even though it is now possible to test your own eyes in some pharmacies and supermarkets to see whether you need reading glasses and what strength of lenses to choose, these d-i-y eye tests are not a substitute for a proper check-up with a professional optician because they are unable to detect other disorders that affect the eye.

You should have your eyes tested at least every two years, particularly over the age of 40, as a slow deterioration in your eyesight will often develop unnoticed. Full eye tests also allow potentially serious, sight-threatening conditions such as glaucoma (see page 224) to be detected and treated before there is any permanent damage. A regular glaucoma test is essential for people who have a close relative (parent or brother/sister) who has suffered from this disorder, as it tends to run in families. In this situation, the eye test will be free after the age of 40. Anyone with a medical condition that can damage the blood vessels at the back of the eyes, for example high blood pressure or diabetes, should have his vision tested at least once a year. Sudden changes in vision, such as seeing coloured haloes around lights, blurring or distortion of images, should be checked out by your doctor or optician as soon as possible.

Hearing tests

Many men wrongly assume that hearing loss is an inevitable part of getting older and can't be treated. Although it is true that as you grow older your hearing mechanism becomes less sensitive to high-frequency sounds, making conversations slightly more difficult to follow, deafness should always be checked out by your doctor.

There may be a simple cause like a build-up of wax in the ear canals, or fluid behind the eardrums. Even when there is a fault in the complex hearing mechanism inside the inner ear, your doctor can arrange hearing tests at the local ear, nose and throat (ENT) clinic to determine the pattern, type and severity of the deafness and to establish whether a hearing aid would be beneficial.

Visiting the dentist

Many men avoid going to the dentist because they wrongly believe that the more they go, the more likely they are to have unnecessary treatment. Nowadays, however, most dentists are much more conservative in their approach, their main aim being to preserve the health of your teeth and gums.

Measures such as scaling and polishing can prevent the onset of tooth decay and gum disease by removing residual plaque and calculus. Dental X-rays may also be taken to reveal cavities and the spread of gum disease causing erosion of the jaw bone. These conditions can then be treated before they cause more serious damage, avoiding the need for more radical procedures.

Medical checks

A thorough medical examination may be required for a number of different reasons, for example before starting a new job, as part of the

TABLE 5

Screening test	Why done?	When recommended?
Weight	To detect excessive weight gain/loss, both of which can harm physical health	Every three years
Blood pressure (BP)	To check condition of heart and circulation	Every five years from age 20 and annually after age 50. Twice a year (at least) if on BP treatment
Urine test	To detect diabetes, kidney disease, urine infection	Every three years. With urinary symptoms, as soon as possible
Blood sugar	To diagnose diabetes	Every 5–10 years, but normally only if you are obese or have a diabetic in your close family
Blood fats (cholesterol)	Risk factor for heart and circulation disease	Every 5–10 years, but normally only if you smoke, have high blood pressure, or someone in your close family has diabetes or heart disease
Bowel screening (sigmoidoscopy and examination of faeces for blood)	To detect bowel cancer	Annual test for men over 50 (controversial). Started at an earlier age in men with ulcerative colitis or if someone in their family had bowel polyps or cancer
Prostate screening: digital rectal examination, ultrasound scan, test for blood level of prostate specific antigen	To detect prostate cancer	No clear recommendation in the UK at present

application for a licence to drive a taxi or heavy goods vehicle, or when taking out a life assurance or personal health insurance policy.

Many men also ask their doctor for a health check because they are seeking reassurance. They may be worried about the effect of their unhealthy lifestyle but reluctant to change their habits; or someone close to them may have been taken ill or died unexpectedly.

It is dangerous, however, to regard a routine medical as a form of MOT certificate, in other words, as a clean bill of health that lasts a year. Only certain medical disorders will be picked up by even the most thorough physical examination and range of tests. And if you continue to follow an unhealthy lifestyle, you are unlikely to stay in good physical condition.

The list of recommended screening procedures in Table 5 includes only those examinations and tests which can reliably diagnose a disorder at an early stage, normally before it has caused any symptoms, and where early treatment increases the chance of a cure or of preventing the development of complications.

Immunisation

Immunisation is not just for children. Adults may be advised to have some or all of the following:

Influenza Annual 'flu jabs are recommended for anyone likely to become seriously ill or to develop complications during an attack of 'flu. This includes people over the age of 65, or individuals of any age who are suffering from a chest, heart or kidney condition, or who are receiving treatment which suppresses their immune system. 'Flu jabs are also given to groups working in an institution, such as teachers and nurses, to reduce the chance of staff shortages during a 'flu epidemic.

Tetanus A full course of three jabs is recommended for all adults who have not been vaccinated before, consisting of two doses four weeks apart and a third dose six months later. Tetanus boosters are recommended at least every ten years, with the first two boosters given routinely and any subsequent booster at the time of a deep or dirty wound, particularly one contaminated by soil, in which tetanus spores live.

Hepatitis A   This type of liver infection is on the increase; a new vaccine which gives long-term protection may be recommended for health-care workers, food handlers, sewage workers, male homosexuals, intravenous drug users and travellers to certain high-risk countries.

Hepatitis B   This serious liver infection, which can cause cancer of the liver in later life, is passed on through contact with contaminated blood or other body fluids; it is far more contagious than the AIDS virus, although it may be transmitted from one person to another in similar ways.

Immunisation against hepatitis B is recommended for health-care workers, male homosexuals, intravenous drug users and family contacts or sexual partners of anyone with this infection. Police officers and prison warders are also advised to request this vaccine because of the relatively high incidence of hepatitis B among criminals, combined with the high risk of being injured at work.

Tuberculosis (TB)   The incidence of tuberculosis is on the increase again. Adults who have not received a BCG vaccination in the past should have a skin test to check their immunity (which could have developed as the result of previous exposure) before immunisation is carried out.

Polio   Assuming the recommended immunisation against polio was completed in childhood, a booster dose is needed every ten years to maintain immunity. There have been two recent cases of polio in fathers exposed to the virus as the result of contact with faeces while changing the nappy of their recently immunised babies; parents who are not immune to polio should therefore be immunised at the same time as their children.

Diphtheria   Any adult who was not immunised against diphtheria in childhood is at risk from this infection and is advised to receive a full course of three injections of low-dose vaccine one month apart.

Travel jabs   Always check with your doctor or travel agent at least two months in advance to find out which immunisations are recommended or compulsory for the countries you will be staying in or passing through. (You can obtain advice by ringing the Health Advice for Travellers★ number.)

Alcohol, smoking and drug abuse

Drinking too much

For most men, drinking alcohol is a pleasant experience and an important part of their social life. Because alcohol can help make you feel more relaxed, comfortable and sociable, it is not surprising that millions of men in the UK drink it on a regular basis.

Despite its social acceptability, however, it is important to remember that alcohol is still a drug and a highly addictive one at that. The more alcohol you drink and the more frequently you drink, the greater the risk of becoming psychologically or physically dependent on alcohol. There is a very fine dividing line between someone who drinks socially and someone who actually needs to drink every day to avoid unpleasant withdrawal symptoms.

Heavy drinkers are aware that over-indulgence can have unpleasant short-term consequences in the form of a terrible hangover the following day, but most do not realise how destructive regular alcohol abuse can be to their long-term physical health.

Drinking alcohol regularly is associated with an increased tolerance to its effects: the body adapts to the continual presence of alcohol so that you have to consume a lot more to notice any change in the way you feel. However, just because a heavy drinker no longer appears to be getting drunk doesn't mean that the large quantities of alcohol being taken in aren't causing serious damage to his body.

Alcohol in excess can be harmful to many different organs and tissues over a period of several years:

- brain – loss of memory, intellectual deterioration, depression and eventually dementia
- skin – persistent facial flushing as a result of blood-vessel damage
- heart and circulation – increased risk of high blood pressure, heart attacks and stroke
- liver – cirrhosis, hepatitis and even liver cancer
- digestive system – gastritis, pancreatitis, peptic ulcer and cancer of the mouth, throat or oesophagus
- nerves – temporary or permanent numbness, tingling and weakness
- sex organs – infertility due to sperm damage, or impotence due to hormonal changes.

WARNING SYMPTOMS OF ALCOHOL ABUSE

- drinking to relieve anxiety or to lift depression
- feeling uncomfortable on going all day without a drink
- lying or feeling guilty about your drinking
- missing work or an appointment through drinking
- drinking more when friends have had enough
- arguing or fighting under the influence of alcohol
- loss of memory, or an attack of the shakes the next day
- intense craving for a drink.

How to reduce your alcohol consumption

There are a number of ways to cut down your consumption of alcohol:

- set yourself a limit before starting and stick to it; learn to say no
- begin with a long soft drink to quench your thirst
- alternate alcoholic and non-alcoholic drinks
- have a mixer such as lemonade or tonic to dilute your drinks
- sip, do not gulp; appreciate the flavour of your drink
- switch to alcohol-free or low-alcohol wines or beers
- keep a diary to identify when and where most of your drinking takes place.
- aim for two alcohol-free days each week; you may need to avoid drinking partners and places on those days

Safe alcohol limits

Alcohol is unlikely to harm your health if you drink only small amounts and avoid drinking every day. In fact, alcohol in moderation, for example an average of one glass of wine per day, has been shown to be good for your heart and circulation, with a protective effect against heart attacks and angina.

The risks of alcohol, described above, are associated with drinking large quantities regularly over several years. Doctors recommend that men should keep their daily intake of alcohol below three to four units, to avoid damaging their health.

A unit of alcohol, roughly equivalent to eight grams, represents half a pint of ordinary beer or lager, one glass of table wine, one small glass of sherry or one single pub measure of spirits. Remember, however, that some real ales and extra-strength lagers contain up to two-and-a-half times as much alcohol as ordinary beer or lager, that fortified wine such as port contains up to twice as much alcohol as ordinary wine and that when you are serving spirits at home you are probably a lot more generous than the pub when it comes to pouring a measure. Cider ranges from between one-and-a-half to two units for a half-pint depending on its strength.

Getting help for an alcohol problem

Unfortunately, most men who are abusing alcohol are either unaware that they have a problem or refuse to admit it. If you or someone close to you is drinking in excess, the first point of contact should be your family doctor or the local branch of Alcoholics Anonymous.★ While it is not possible to force someone to go for treatment, it is worth trying to reason with the person at a time when he is sober. Alcoholics Anonymous offers advice and guidance for people with a drink problem and provides support to the whole family (try also AL-ANON).★ In severe cases, it may be necessary to admit an alcoholic to hospital for a period of detoxification, with medication prescribed to control the unpleasant withdrawal symptoms.

Long-term treatment to prevent a return to previous drinking habits can include behavioural therapy and psychotherapy; occasionally, a drug known as disulfuram is prescribed, which induces unpleasant side-effects when taken with alcohol.

Smoking – more than just a cancer risk

Cigarette smoking is the most important self-inflicted cause of illness and premature death in Western countries. Smoking has been directly linked with cancers of the lung, mouth, throat, larynx, oesophagus and bladder. In addition, smokers appear to have a higher risk of cancers of the pancreas, kidney and stomach.

While most men are aware of the cancer risk from smoking, there are also many other less well-publicised smoking-related diseases. A smoker's cough may progress to chronic bronchitis and emphysema, causing breathlessness severe enough to stop someone leading a normal lifestyle. Smokers also have a much greater chance of suffering from angina, heart attacks or a stroke, or of needing an amputation because of blocked circulation in one or more of their limbs. Evidence also suggests that regular smoking can result in shrinking of the penis.

It is generally never too late to benefit from giving up smoking. For example, the risk of premature death from a heart attack or chronic bronchitis is almost halved within five years of quitting tobacco.

How to give up smoking

Nearly four out of every five smokers say they would like to quit, encouraged by the knowledge that they would almost certainly improve their life expectancy and their quality of life. However, the fact that only about one-quarter of those who try manage to give up demonstrates how powerfully addictive the smoking habit is. Quitline★ offers advice to smokers who want to give up.

To improve your chance of quitting successfully, try to identify the reasons why you smoke. Then you can adopt the tactics best suited to the type of smoker you are.

The nicotine addict Smokers who suffer unpleasant withdrawal symptoms, such as headaches, anxiety, irritability and an intense craving for a cigarette can benefit from a nicotine substitute in the form of skin patches, a nasal spray, an inhalator (which is like a cigarette without the toxins) or chewing gum. Ask your doctor or pharmacist for advice and counselling on how best to use nicotine-replacement therapy.

Smoking to socialise This type of smoker should avoid the places where he will be tempted or encouraged to smoke and keep away from friends who will continue to offer him cigarettes.

Smoking to relieve tension Use other techniques to reduce stress, such as a new hobby, playing sport or learning a relaxation exercise (see Chapter 3).

Smoking to occupy hands and mouth Chew sugar-free gum to keep your mouth busy, play with worry beads to distract your fingers.

Smoking to fight boredom Become interested in a new activity, preferably one that occupies your hands, such as learning to play the guitar or model-making.

Smoking as a routine   At those times when you invariably light up a cigarette, for example after a meal, do something else instead.

EXTRA TIPS ON GIVING UP

- make a list of all your reasons for quitting
- choose a time when you are not going to be highly stressed
- stop abruptly at a set time; cutting down gradually rarely works
- give up with a friend who can offer extra support
- throw away cigarettes, lighters, ashtrays etc.
- avoid chocolate, red meat, tea, coffee and alcohol, which can all increase craving
- drink plenty of water, fruit juice and herbal tea
- spend the money you save on cigarettes on something special
- consider hypnosis or acupuncture if you are having difficulty stopping.

Weight gain

Some men find that they put on a few kilograms in weight after they give up smoking. This is partly because they are no longer taking in nicotine, which stimulates the body's metabolism, and partly because their appetite will tend to increase as a result of better awareness of taste. However, if you only nibble on healthy snacks (see page 65), you are unlikely to put on more than a few kilograms, and being a little overweight is nowhere near as bad for your health as continuing to smoke.

Drug abuse – the risks

A wide variety of drugs may be misused, including some drugs normally prescribed by a doctor, such as painrelievers, stimulants, tranquillisers and anabolic steroids. In such cases, they are often taken in amounts far in excess of the normal dosage. Other drugs that are commonly misused, such as cannabis, Ecstasy, LSD, amphetamine, cocaine and crack cocaine, are either home-grown, manufactured illicitly in home laboratories, or illegally imported from abroad.

There are many different reasons for abusing drugs, including the desire to escape from reality, the search for self-awareness, trying to achieve a mystical experience, or simply a curiosity about the effects.

Amphetamines and anabolic steroids are sometimes abused in an attempt to improve sporting performance.

Regular or excessive use of a drug may lead to addiction, either in the form of psychological dependence, in which the individual experiences severe emotional distress or intense craving when that drug is no longer being taken, or physical dependence, in which stopping the drug abruptly results in unpleasant withdrawal symptoms that may last several days.

Tolerance to a drug may also develop with regular usage, which will make it necessary to use progressively larger amounts of the drug to achieve the same effect. Drug dependence almost inevitably leads to a deterioration in physical as well as emotional health, in addition to the financial problems related to paying for the habit and probably becoming unfit for work.

Tranquillisers (e.g. benzodiazepines) Nowadays, doctors generally prescribe these drugs only for short periods in as low a dosage as possible. Regular use for more than two weeks is likely to lead to physical dependence. After long-term prescription, the dose of benzodiazepine has to be reduced gradually over several weeks to avoid unpleasant withdrawal symptoms. Due to their calming, relaxing effect, benzodiazepines are commonly abused, particularly by people abusing other drugs, such as opiates and stimulants.

Barbiturates These sedative drugs are still prescribed for epilepsy and occasionally for insomnia. Like benzodiazepines, a barbiturate may be abused for its relaxing, calming effect. Regular use leads to physical dependence and accidental overdose can be fatal if it stops the normal breathing mechanism.

Opiate drugs These narcotic painrelievers, which include heroin, morphine and dihydrocodeine, are used medically to treat severe pain. They are abused because of their ability to induce a state of euphoria. Regular misuse of an opiate leads to physical dependence and accidental overdose can cause coma and death if the breathing mechanism is suppressed.

Amphetamines These stimulant drugs, which were once commonly prescribed as appetite suppressants, are abused to induce feelings of excitement and boost energy levels, particularly by individuals who are suffering the effects of fatigue or lack of sleep. Regular amphetamine abuse can result in paranoia or aggressive behaviour. An overdose may cause palpitations, hallucinations, a dangerous rise in blood pressure and, on rare occasions, seizures.

Ecstasy ('E') This powerful stimulant, chemically similar to amphetamine, has become popular among young people. Although many have taken this drug with no apparent ill effects, there have been several deaths and a number of serious adverse psychiatric and physical reactions as a result of the action of this drug on the brain, heart, muscles and other parts of the body. When Ecstasy is used at parties or 'raves' the chance of heat exhaustion and dehydration may be reduced by wearing loose cotton clothing and drinking regular, moderate amounts of non-alcoholic fluids.

Potentially fatal toxic effects from Ecstasy have included seizures, hepatitis, kidney failure and a dangerous increase in body temperature. Risks are greater when large numbers of Ecstasy tablets are taken at once or if the tablets have been adulterated with other drugs, such as amphetamine and LSD, or other harmful substances.

LSD This powerful hallucinogenic drug, which was once used in psychiatric patients receiving psychotherapy, produces unpredictable effects with bizarre hallucinations that may be pleasant or terrifying. Several people have died while under the influence of LSD, for example, by trying to fly from an upper floor window and, occasionally, a single dose leads to prolonged psychosis in a vulnerable individual.

Cocaine This drug, originally obtained from the leaves of plants growing naturally in South America, is now also produced synthetically. Its rapid numbing action on the skin and mucous membrane surfaces, which lasts for up to an hour, made cocaine an ideal anaesthetic for minor surgical procedures involving the eye, ear, nose or throat. Because it also narrows blood vessels, its anaesthetic effect remains localised.

Absorbed into the main bloodstream, however, cocaine interferes with normal brain chemistry to induce feelings of increased energy, well-being, elation and euphoria. This has led to widespread abuse of cocaine, usually by inhalation through the nose (snorting). As a result of this abuse potential, doctors have switched to using other types of local anaesthetic.

Regular snorting of cocaine powder can damage the lining of the nose, causing uncomfortable congestion in the short term and, eventually, total tissue destruction, with perforation of the nasal septum. People who regularly abuse cocaine are likely to become psychologically dependent on it, experiencing intense cravings for the next high. Large doses may cause a psychotic reaction, seizures or cardiac arrest.

Crack cocaine Crack is a purified form of cocaine made by a process known as free-basing to produce small rocks about the size of raisins. Smoking crack induces a much more intense and rapid psychological effect than sniffing cocaine powder, with extreme euphoria and a sense of heightened physical and mental capacity. However, these feelings wear off within about 12 minutes typically leaving the user severely anxious or depressed, with loss of appetite and difficulty in sleeping. Frequent doses are therefore required to sustain a high. Regular crack smoking may cause a chronic cough, wheeze and a partial loss of voice. Long-standing abuse also leads to suicidal feelings, unpredictable behaviour, delusions and hallucinations. As with cocaine powder, a crack overdose can result in seizures and cardiac arrest.

Marijuana This popular recreational drug comes from the flowering tops and dried leaves of the Indian hemp plant *Cannabis sativa*. It is used for its ability to cause euphoria, enhanced perception, feelings of relaxation and pleasant drowsiness, with time seeming to pass more slowly. The lack of physical and psychological problems associated with marijuana has led to a national campaign to legalise it. However, it may aggravate or unmask a psychiatric condition in someone who was already at risk and is known to impair short-term memory.

Giving up marijuana after regular use does not produce unpleasant withdrawal symptoms, but persistent use may cause apathy or depression. There is also concern about the influence marijuana may have on driving, due to its effect on visuo-spatial judgement, but this has not been supported by accident statistics.

Individuals who smoke marijuana with tobacco, rather than on its own, are exposed to all the health risks associated with cigarette smoking (see page 97–8).

Solvents   More than 100 domestic products, including glue and cleaning fluid, may be deliberately inhaled to induce euphoria or hallucinations. Continued inhalation can rapidly lead to drowsiness, loss of co-ordination, slurred speech and disorientation. Severe intoxication occasionally results in seizures, coma and death. Other risks include asphyxia during inhalation and accidents occurring while under the influence of the solvent. Long-term toxic effects from regular solvent abuse include brain, liver and kidney damage.

Anabolic steroids   These drugs regularly hit the headlines when an athlete or sportsperson is found to have traces of anabolic steroid in his or her urine. The reason for abusing this type of drug is to boost the development of strong, bulky muscles. By speeding up the recovery of muscles after a strenuous workout in the gym, anabolic steroids allow a more demanding training programme. Most authorities governing the various competitive sports have banned the use of anabolic steroids, not only because they confer an unfair advantage, but also due to their potential to cause serious side-effects, such as liver damage and infertility.

Overcoming drug addiction

If you or someone close to you has become dependent on any drug, the first step is to seek professional help through, for example, your family doctor or by contacting an organisation such as Release* or the Standing Conference on Drug Abuse (SCODA).* The addict will usually be referred to a specialised drug rehabilitation centre, where a gradual withdrawal from the substance can be followed through under careful medical supervision.

Once a drug habit has been overcome, professional counselling, psychotherapy or behaviour therapy may be recommended to help prevent a relapse. Self-help groups can assist motivation to stay off drugs; it is also crucial to break with drug-taking friends, to move to new surroundings and to form new relationships.

Chapter 3

Coping with stress

MANY men thrive on stress; they are unhappy unless there are deadlines to meet and more than one job on the go at any one time. A performer on stage or an athlete in competition will often find the inherent stress exhilarating. The way in which you handle stress is determined partly by your personality and partly by your innate ability to cope under different types of pressure. However, there is also a great deal you can do to enable stress to work for you, rather than work against you.

Stress under control can be a positive force that improves performance, provides stimulation and motivation and keeps you on your toes and out of danger. Some degree of stress is essential to add spice to your life and prevent you from becoming bored and apathetic.

All men experience intense stress at certain times in their life, for example, when circumstances suddenly change or an event beyond their control occurs. However, stress overload increases the risk of both mental and physical illnesses, as well as increasing susceptibility to accidental injuries. Over half of all visits to the doctor are thought to be related in some way to stress, usually in the form of worries about work or money.

Causes of stress

Stress is triggered by an activity or circumstance that arouses the emotions or is perceived to be a threat or danger. This includes a wide variety of stimuli: for example, being on the receiving end of verbal or physical aggression; a traumatic life event such as losing your job or moving house; or an internal conflict, such as guilt.

All these stressful situations cause characteristic physical changes in the body, which represent a primitive reaction to stress that enabled our ancestors either to fight or to escape from everyday dangers ('fight or flight'). This response occurs as a result of the release of stress hormones – adrenaline, noradrenaline and cortisol – from the activated adrenal glands and stimulation of the sympathetic nerves around the body. Physical changes brought on by stress prepare the body to perform to maximum efficiency:

- heart beats stronger and more rapidly
- breathing becomes deeper and faster
- muscles receive greater blood flow
- sweating increases to prevent overheating
- pupils widen to let in more light; eyes focus for distance vision
- blood sugar levels rise to provide an energy source for muscles.

Harmful effects of stress

Ideally, stress is a temporary condition that arises to meet a specific challenge and subsides once those demands have been resolved. After a short period of stress, the body is then allowed to return to its resting state. Problems arise when:

- the threat is mental or emotional rather than physical, in which case the 'fight or flight' response is unhelpful. Changes, such as a more rapid heartbeat, increased muscle tension and sweating, do not provide a defence against psychological pressure and there is no opportunity to work off your arousal through physical exertion
- the threat is prolonged, for example, constant pressure from a demanding job or an unhappy relationship. People who are unable to escape from or conquer their source of stress remain in a heightened state of arousal and the result of this continuous and unwanted tension is likely to be an adverse effect on both mental and physical health.

Stressful life events

Some people find even relatively minor irritations like a queue at a ticket office or being held up in a traffic jam stressful, while others are able to stay calm and relaxed. There are, however, a number of traumatic life events that cause great stress for almost everyone: for example, the death of your partner, being sent to jail, divorce, losing your job, impending fatherhood.

Although a particular change in his life may cause more stress for one man than for another, it is still possible to predict the risk of stress-related illness from the number and nature of life events which an individual has been through.

Warning symptoms

Many men are unaware of just how much stress they are under. They fail to recognise the early-warning symptoms of stress overload. It is only when you acknowledge the harmful levels of stress in your life that you will be able to do something positive to protect your emotional and physical health.

Common symptoms of stress include:

- difficulty falling asleep
- inability to concentrate or make decisions
- increasing irritability, impatience and loss of temper
- constantly feeling tired or lethargic
- eating when not hungry
- smoking more, drinking more alcohol
- recurrent headaches, muscle or joint pains
- reduced interest in sex
- driving fast and dangerously.

Stress-related illness

Almost every illness has some link with your state of mind and your emotions; feeling depressed can make a physical condition seem a lot more serious than it really is. The term 'psychosomatic' is used to describe any illness that appears to have been caused or aggravated by psychological factors. This does not mean that a psychosomatic illness is imaginary, simply that emotional problems are a major influence on the condition. Common disorders that are sometimes, but not always, psychosomatic include irritable bowel syndrome and tension headaches. Anyone who has suffered from these conditions will know just how genuine the symptoms are.

Prolonged minor stresses or a source of intense stress may contribute to a variety of disorders affecting different parts of the body:

- skin – eczema and psoriasis may both flare up during times of stress
- reproductive organs – stress is the most common cause of impotence and premature ejaculation

- digestive system – stress-related problems include gastritis, peptic ulcer, irritable bowel and colitis
- immune system – stress is known to increase susceptibility to infection
- heart and circulation – stress can increase blood pressure, which in turn raises the risk of suffering a heart attack or stroke
- lungs – emotional upset may aggravate some cases of asthma
- hair – baldness is occasionally brought on by extreme stress
- brain – stress may be the cause of many mental and emotional problems, such as anxiety and depression. The popular term 'nervous breakdown' refers to a stress-related condition in which the individual is no longer able to deal with everyday problems.

Coping with stress

While it is clearly impossible, as well as undesirable, to avoid stress altogether, there is a lot you can do to improve your ability to cope with stressful situations and prevent stress overload. First, you need to recognise the early-warning symptoms of stress, as described above. Then you should attempt to identify the various sources of stress in your life and decide what you are going to do about them. Any action you take to relieve stress is bound to do some good because it is an indication that you are no longer prepared to put up with this unacceptable level of pressure.

If you are having trouble pinpointing the exact cause of your stress, make a note of the circumstances each time you start to feel more anxious and see whether a pattern emerges. The key to reducing stress is to deal with one problem at a time. Make a list, in order of priority, and start with the situation that is causing the most distress, leaving the minor irritations to last.

Talk frankly to anyone you see as being at the root of your troubles. Admitting that things are getting on top of you may be an awkward or embarrassing confession to make to your partner, your children, your parents or your boss. The sooner you involve the other person, however, the sooner you will be able to find a constructive solution.

It is also important to express your emotions openly, rather than trying to bottle them up. Don't be afraid to show that you are angry or sad; crying doesn't reflect a loss of masculinity, nor does it mean you will lose the respect of those around you.

There are other ways to keep your stress levels under control:

- where possible, avoid making too many changes in your life at once
- don't brood about situations or events over which you have no control
- don't feel guilty about having to change arrangements or ideas
- cultivate your social life – all work and no play damages health
- exercise regularly to release pent-up emotions, reduce tension, take your mind off any particular worries and encourage deep, refreshing sleep
- use a regular relaxation technique, such as breathing exercises, muscle relaxation, meditation, yoga or massage.

If you are unable to sort out your stress-related problems on your own using the self-help measures and relaxation techniques described in this chapter, do not delay going to see your doctor, particularly if you feel the stress in your life is out of control, making you feel ill, or preventing you from leading a normal life. You may need counselling to help you adjust your outlook or lifestyle. If your emotional disorder is severe, you may need medication, for example to lift your depression or suppress your anxiety.

Managing stress at home

Stress in the home is often more intense than many people realise, with a wide variety of potential problems straining the emotional health of each family member. The father, for example, may be put under increased stress by the arrival of a new baby, his daughter leaving home, his wife going back to work, the death of one of his parents. His response to these events and the way the rest of the family responds add up to a complex mix of stresses. Different families will be affected in different ways, and some will handle the situation a lot better than others.

The best way to cope during and after any period of domestic stress is to allow everyone in the family to communicate their feelings and fears as far as possible. It is also essential to try to appreciate the stress other family members are under.

Remember that the person who stays at home to look after the children is not taking the easy option. Running a home and raising children is a full-time occupation which is usually highly stressful; many women do this and a paid job as well.

Many parents do not realise just how much stress their children are putting them under and wrongly feel guilty if they lose patience with them. A child may continually demand attention and, if one or both parents' sleep is being regularly disturbed, he or she is likely to end up exhausted and irritable. Ways to cope with this type of stress are discussed in detail in Chapter 5.

If money worries are a major factor behind the build-up of stress in your home, contact your bank or a financial adviser for help. Do not make the mistake of just ignoring all the people you owe money to – banks and building societies are much more sympathetic if you explain your situation, and can help you organise a system of repayment.

When someone in the family is violent or has an alcohol or drug problem, the resultant pressures in the home will put all the family members at risk of stress-related illness. In this situation it is vital to seek professional help, starting with your GP or the Samaritans.★

Marriage breakdown

One in three marriages in the UK ends in divorce and second marriages are even less likely to work. Warning symptoms that your relationship with your partner is under threat include:

- difficulty talking about personal problems
- frequent arguments or fits of temper which you then regret
- intense jealousy
- believing you are contributing a lot more than your partner
- feeling trapped or held back
- no longer looking forward to coming home
- an unsatisfying sex life with your partner
- a desire for other sexual relationships.

Holidays are a common time for relationship difficulties to come to the surface. Couples wrongly expect everything to be fine away from the pressures of work; but, in reality, the holiday takes them away from the activities they were using to avoid each other and forces them to confront their conflicting attitudes and emotions.

Saving your relationship

Married couples or established partners who are going through a bad patch in their relationship, which they have been unable to sort out themselves, often benefit from professional counselling. For some couples, however, divorce or separation provides a welcome release from the stress of living with an incompatible partner.

You can make an appointment with one of the counsellors employed by the national organisation Relate★ (formerly the Marriage Guidance Council). Alternatively, you can see your GP, who may be trained in counselling, or you may be referred to a clinical psychologist who specialises in marital problems.

Partners should attend the counselling sessions together on a regular basis. Marital therapy begins with an analysis of the good and bad aspects of the relationship, with both parties encouraged to express openly their grievances and how they would like to see an improvement. Any blame for the marriage/relationship problems should be shared equally.

In addition to learning to communicate more effectively with each other, couples should try to find a leisure activity that they can both enjoy together. Sex therapy may also be recommended, although any problems with a sexual relationship will only be resolved once difficulties outside the bedroom have been overcome.

Stress management at work

If you feel under stress as a result of your job, try to identify which of the following reasons apply to your situation at work:

- no control over your workload
- recently passed over for promotion
- threat of redundancy
- too much/not enough responsibility
- working long hours
- having to take work home
- excessive competition
- hostility from colleagues
- sexual harassment (see page 112)
- unrealistic deadlines
- no procedure to settle grievances
- enforced relocation to a new area
- boredom
- job dissatisfaction
- working only for the money

- difficult or uncomfortable journey to and from work
- demotion
- unwanted promotion
- conflict of loyalties
- unpleasant confrontation with the public.

If nothing is done to resolve your problems at work you are likely to become ill. The symptoms may be back pain or depression, but the real reason is job-related stress.

Changing your approach

Many men could regain control of the stress related to their work by managing their time more effectively and taking regular time out to relax and unwind. To improve your time-management skills, stick to the following principles – you will soon notice an improvement both in your productivity and the way you feel about your job.

- It is important not to waste time procrastinating. Prepare a list of the tasks you need to accomplish in order of priority. Set yourself realistic goals and say no to unreasonable demands and impracticable deadlines. Finish one job before you move on to the next.
- Divide large projects into more manageable chunks and delegate work to others when you can.
- Take regular breaks during the day. A brief rest period will help refresh your mind after a long session of concentrated mental effort and stop you becoming frustrated with a project. It is best to go for a change in scenery, for example, by taking a walk in a nearby park, if possible.
- Transfer any uncompleted task to the following day's action plan and make a note of anything that interfered with your work schedule which you may be able to rectify; it may be necessary, for example, to have someone take phone messages for part of the day to avoid constant interruptions.
- Take weekend breaks and proper holidays, preferably away from home, to prevent you getting stuck into potentially stressful activities like clearing out the garage.

Clearly some of the problems listed at the beginning of this section cannot be solved simply by changing your approach to work. Ideally, you should communicate your difficulties either directly to your boss or indirectly via your union or staff committee. However, you should be aware of the need to handle the situation tactfully to avoid being seen as a troublemaker.

If you decide to try your hand at something different, think about gaining extra qualifications in your spare time before putting in your notice. Men stuck in a bad job situation should concentrate on achieving fulfilment and enjoyment from their life outside of work.

SEXUAL HARASSMENT

It is not just women who get sexually harassed; men may be harassed by women or other men at work.

If this is happening to you, try to avoid contact with the individual as far as possible, although this may be difficult within the confines of an office or shop floor. Be assertive by making it clear that you find this behaviour offensive, but there is no need to be rude.

If the situation doesn't improve, you will need to make a formal complaint. In the meantime, keep a detailed diary of each episode of harassment and the circumstances in which it occurred as this will help you prepare your case. Also, discreetly ask your male colleagues whether they have been experiencing the same problem.

Relaxation techniques

Relaxation is a skill that everyone should learn because it is an essential part of a healthy lifestyle. It doesn't matter which of the many techniques you choose to help you relax, but you should practise regularly to gain the maximum benefit for your physical and emotional health. Regular use of a relaxation technique will also make it easier for you to cope during periods of more intense stress. In addition to reducing muscle tension, daily relaxation will help relieve stress-related conditions, such as recurrent headaches and back pain.

Breathing exercise

Try the following exercise for five minutes at a time twice a day and then use it whenever you start to feel tense or anxious:

- find a quiet area where you won't be disturbed by people or the telephone
- sit in a comfortable chair with your feet flat on the floor, relax your shoulders and become aware of the chair supporting you
- consciously slow your rate of breathing and take deep, even breaths
- breathe out for twice as long as you breathe in, controlling this pattern by silently counting to yourself
- during this breathing exercise, try to clear your mind of all thoughts and worries
- stop deep breathing if you begin to feel dizzy.

Muscle relaxation

Muscles that have become tense and taut can be relaxed by the following simple routine. Find somewhere that is quiet, warm and dimly lit where you won't be disturbed; take off your shoes and remove any spectacles or contact lenses before you begin. Ideally, you should be wearing comfortable, loose-fitting clothing which allows you to move each part of your body freely.

- lie flat on your back either on a bed or the floor
- close your eyes, let all your muscles go limp and breathe at your normal resting rate and rhythm
- tighten the muscles in your toes for a few seconds before relaxing them as you breathe out
- work up your body, tightening and then relaxing each group of muscles in turn
- when you reach your face, screw up the muscles around your mouth and eyes, then let them relax as if the skin on your face is sliding off on to the floor
- raise your head for a few seconds, then relax your neck and jaw muscles to allow your head to fall gently back and your mouth and throat to open
- repeat this whole toe-to-head sequence until ten minutes have passed, then lie completely still for a few more minutes; you should feel totally relaxed
- stretch your arms and legs gently before going back into action.

Meditation

Traditionally, meditation has been an integral part of many different religions, particularly those based on Eastern philosophies. People experienced in meditation often use these techniques as a pathway towards spiritual awareness and fulfilment. For most people in the West, however, the aim of meditation is simply to release inner tension and achieve a state of deep relaxation by emptying the mind of distracting thoughts and worries.

A variety of organisations teach meditation. The most common form practised in the West is transcendental meditation (TM)*, in which the individual is given a personal secret word or sound (a *mantra*) by the instructor to say over and over again to himself.

To see if meditation works for you, try the following simple exercise. Find a quiet room where you won't be disturbed and try to sit cross-legged with your back straight, but modify this position as necessary to get comfortable. Breathe at your normal resting rate and rhythm, close your eyes and choose one of these techniques to empty your mind of thoughts and ideas:

- repeat a word or phrase silently to yourself without moving your lips; the word or words should have no emotional significance so you can concentrate on the exercise itself and not think about the meaning
- imagine a beautiful scene and savour every minute detail of this picture in your mind's eye
- alternatively, with your eyes open, stare at one specific stationary object such as the pattern on a wall, but don't attempt to analyse its form or shape.

Meditate for only five minutes at a time until you find it easier to clear your mind of distractions. With practice, you will gradually be able to increase your session of meditation up to a maximum of 20 minutes.

Whichever technique you follow, you will find that your mind wanders, or distracting thoughts start to intrude. The trick is to take yourself gently back to concentrating on your word, phrase, image or object each time this happens. There is no need to actively force out these distractions, simply try not to follow them and not to worry about how well you are doing.

Yoga

Although yoga is based on an ancient system of Indian philosophy and physical discipline, this activity has become increasingly popular in the West in recent decades. Not only is yoga a useful relaxation technique that helps calm the mind and reduce tension, some exercises produce physical benefits, including helping to improve flexibility, balance and co-ordination, and increasing muscle strength and endurance.

It is best to learn yoga in a supervised class. In Hatha yoga you will be taught co-ordinated movements and postures, called *asanas*, that exercise virtually every part of your body, combined with breath-control techniques known as *pranayamas*. In Siddha yoga the emphasis is on meditation techniques.

People who experiment with Hatha yoga on their own run the risk of over-stretching injuries. Elderly people and anyone with a specific medical disorder such as high blood pressure, back trouble or glaucoma (raised pressure in the eye – see page 224) may have to avoid or modify certain positions. (The Yoga for Health Foundation* and the British Wheel of Yoga* can offer advice.)

Massage

Thanks to the sex industry, massage has acquired a somewhat sleazy reputation. However, there are many *bona fide* massage practitioners who are experienced in massage techniques that have nothing to do with sexual stimulation. There are also several good books available which will teach you how to massage your partner and yourself.

Massage involves stroking, kneading and pummelling the muscles and other soft tissues in various parts of the body. It is a powerful relaxation technique which is tremendously comforting, producing a positive feeling of well-being in both the recipient and the person giving the massage. A foot massage not only makes your feet feel good, but also refreshes and relaxes your whole body. A facial massage can relieve tension headaches and stress-related fatigue, as well as leaving your face looking and feeling fresher and younger.

Massage is available only in a few GPs' surgeries and hospital clinics, so most people will have to go for private treatment. Because anyone can set themselves up as a massage practitioner, without any experience or qualifications, it is advisable to visit only a chartered physiotherapist (with the letters MCSP) who offers massage therapy, or someone approved by the Federation of Holistic Therapists.*

MASSAGE SAFETY TIPS

Do not eat or drink immediately before a massage. Tense muscles may feel uncomfortable during a massage, but you should not feel sore afterwards.

Massage is not recommended for those with any of the following conditions:

- a fever or infection, including skin infection
- skin inflammation in the area to be massaged
- pain made worse or spread to other areas when pressure is applied
- thrombosis, phlebitis or varicose veins (may be aggravated by massage of the affected area).

Teach yourself massage

There is no substitute for practical tuition in the art of massage. However, here are some basic tips to get you started:

- choose a warm, dimly lit, quiet room where you won't be disturbed
- remove anything that might scratch, irritate or be distracting, such as a watch or bracelet; rings should be removed or covered with tape
- only the area being massaged should be exposed: cover the rest of the body with towels
- assuming you do not have a specialised massage couch, the person being massaged should lie on a firm padded surface, most likely a bed. If the bed does not have a firm mattress, use blankets, foam rubber or a mattress on the floor; the masseur or masseuse should kneel on something comfortable
- to enable your hands to glide smoothly over the skin, use a light vegetable oil or talcum powder. A range of aromatherapy massage oils is available, each of which is recommended for specific disorders
- if you use a massage oil, never pour it directly on to the skin of the person being massaged. Put less than one teaspoonful into the palm of your hand and warm the oil up by rubbing your hands together
- start with circular stroking movements, moulding your hands to the contours of the body and keeping to a constant rhythm

- keep one hand in contact with the body at all times. If you need more oil, pour a little on to the back of the massaging hand and continue stroking while you use your free hand to transfer this extra oil lightly on to the skin
- during the massage, concentrate on your hand movements and don't talk too much
- on small areas, stroke with your thumbs or fingertips
- over larger muscles, use firmer pressure but don't push too hard
- if massage is causing a ticklish sensation, increase the pressure or move to a different area
- to release muscle tension, apply deep pressure with your thumbs either kept still or moving in tiny circles
- to relax tense muscles in the fleshy areas around the shoulders, hips and thighs, try a kneading technique. Pummelling with loosely clenched fists with your wrists relaxed will create a light, bouncy pressure on the muscles, which will also help.

Chapter 4

Sexual health and awareness

WHATEVER your sexual orientation, it is important to understand the principles of safer sex and to know about the symptoms and treatment of different sexually transmitted diseases. Also, because sexual arousal and responses are broadly similar in heterosexual and homosexual men, the advice given in this chapter on how to overcome relatively common psychosexual problems, such as impotence and premature ejaculation, is relevant to all men.

No attempt is made here to offer recommendations on how to vary or improve your sex life, a matter beyond the bounds of 'health', but those who want this information will find the subject amply covered in other books and in magazines and educational videos.

Safer sex

Safe sex used to mean taking precautions to avoid an unwanted pregnancy. Nowadays, with the spread of HIV (Human Immunodeficiency Virus) infection and AIDS (Acquired Immune Deficiency Syndrome), this term more commonly refers to precautions taken to protect against sexually transmitted diseases (STDs). However, because absolute protection is impossible, it is more accurate to refer to the practice of *safer* sex.

Despite all the publicity warning of the risk of HIV infection, many heterosexual men – particularly those in their 20s and 30s – do not practise safer sex. One reason for this is that some people still believe that it is only homosexual men and drug addicts who are likely to expose themselves to HIV and AIDS. In 1997, however, there were 343 new cases of HIV infection and 202 new AIDS cases among men in the UK, probably acquired through sexual intercourse with a woman. Another common problem is that while many men agree that using a condom is a good idea, most don't bother in practice. They may carry condoms, but unless their partners insist that they use them, they invariably don't. Although a recent survey by the Health Education Authority (HEA)* revealed that 65 per cent of 16- to 24-year-old men reported that they would use a condom the first time they had sex with a new partner, they are much less likely to continue to use a condom in the early stages of a relationship. In a previous HEA survey, only 30 per cent of 18- to 24-year-old men had used a condom the last time they had sex.

Even more alarming is the fact that the men least likely to use a condom are those who have the most sexual encounters and who therefore run the greatest risk of picking up and passing on sexually transmitted diseases.

A survey of gay men published in 1996 found that one in three reported unprotected anal intercourse with at least one male partner, and one in ten with more than one male partner.

SAFER SEX RECOMMENDATIONS

- When having intercourse (vaginal or anal), you should always use a condom for at least the first three months of a mutually monogamous relationship (anal sex is actually illegal in England, Wales and Northern Ireland between a man and a woman).
- Before stopping the use of condoms, you and your partner should both have a sexual health check-up at your GP's surgery or an STD clinic (see below).
- If both you and your partner are clear of disease and monogamous, there is no need to use a condom, except as a method of contraception (if the relationship is not mutually monogamous, condoms are still required).
- Some STDs can be passed on by oral or anal sex.

STD clinics

If you have symptoms of an STD, or have been with someone suspected or known to have an STD, it is important for you to have a check-up as soon as possible. For most types of STD, the earlier treatment is started, the less likely it is that complications will develop.

However, the STD clinic is not just for people worried about infection; clinic staff can also provide advice about sexual health and encourage both men and women to go for regular check-ups, even if they have no symptoms. A good time for a check-up is before starting a new sexual relationship, or before giving up using condoms with a regular partner.

STD clinics are listed in the telephone directory under STD, VD or genito-urinary (GU) medicine. Alternatively, the local hospital will have a GU or 'special' clinic, which you can call to make an appointment; it is not necessary to be referred by a GP. Some clinics will give you a time for an appointment over the phone, others see patients in the order they arrive. Appointments and treatment at an NHS clinic are free, private STD clinics currently charge about £50–£60, including standard tests.

You may give a false name if you prefer, but your details are completely confidential and will not be revealed to your doctor, employer, insurance company or partner without your permission. STD clinics do provide the Department of Health with information about the number of cases of a particular STD, to keep statistics up to date, but this does not include patient names or any personal details.

Whatever condition you suspect you are suffering from, it is routine practice to screen for all STDs apart from HIV, which is usually tested for only on request and with counselling about the significance of the result. After questions about your sexual habits and any symptoms you might have, your physical examination will normally include a swab being taken from the opening to the urethra at the tip of the penis; urine and blood samples will also be taken.

Some results will be available within a few minutes, but for other tests you need to telephone later or call back in person. It is usually possible for the clinic doctor to make at least a provisional diagnosis and any treatment necessary can be provided straight away.

Although not obliged to let previous or current sexual partners know about any STD you have picked up, the clinic staff will encourage you to give permission for them to get in touch with your sexual contacts. They do not have to give your name to these people; they simply advise them to attend their local clinic for treatment.

Common sexually transmitted diseases

At the beginning of this century the most common STDs were gonorrhoea and syphilis; now it is non-specific urethritis (NSU) that tops the list, along with genital warts and genital herpes. Media attention is focused mainly on HIV and AIDS, but at present the number of known cases of these conditions in the UK is relatively small compared to those of other STDs.

Non-specific urethritis (NSU)

Urethritis is inflammation of the urethra, the narrow tube that runs through the penis carrying either urine from the bladder or semen on ejaculation. The most common cause of urethritis in men, non-specific urethritis (NSU), is due to infection with chlamydia, a type of bug that has some of the characteristics of bacteria and other features that are more typical of viruses.

NSU may cause a burning discomfort on passing urine and a yellowish discharge from the penis. The diagnosis may be confirmed by examining a swab of the discharge under a microscope. Treatment is with a course of antibiotics, usually a type of tetracycline. Left untreated, NSU in men may spread to infect the testicle and epididymis, causing pain, tenderness and swelling. Joint and eye inflammation are other possible complications.

All sexual partners of an NSU sufferer should also be treated with antibiotics, regardless of whether they have noticed any urethral discomfort or discharge. This is because many women who pick up a chlamydia infection remain free of urinary symptoms, or the urethral discharge is masked by their normal vaginal discharge. Men can develop inflammation of the rectum as a complication of NSU, although it may not cause any symptoms.

Gonorrhoea

Symptoms of gonorrhoea may appear at any time between two and ten days after exposure to this bacterial infection, with a discharge of pus from the urethra and pain on passing urine that can vary from a mild discomfort to a severe burning sensation. Oral sex with someone who is infected with gonorrhoea can lead to painful inflammation of the throat. Gonorrhoea picked up by anal sex can result in anal irritation and discharge due to inflammation of the rectum.

Examination under the microscope of swabs taken from the urethra and, when necessary, from the throat and rectum, will confirm the diagnosis. Treatment with antibiotics is usually effective and should be given to all sexual partners. Left untreated, gonorrhoea may spread to infect the testicles or prostate gland. Arthritis and blood poisoning are other possible complications.

Trichomoniasis

This STD is caused by a single-cell parasite, which may invade and multiply inside the urethra and under the foreskin (in uncircumcised men), occasionally spreading to the prostate gland. Symptoms of trichomoniasis in men may include discomfort on passing urine and a yellowish-green urethral discharge. Many men who are exposed to this infection do not have symptoms and there is no discharge to examine for parasites under the microscope. Nevertheless, if your female sexual partner has been diagnosed as suffering from trichomoniasis you should be treated with the antibiotic metronidazole to avoid the risk of re-infecting her in the future.

Thrush

This common yeast infection may be passed on through sexual intercourse with an infected partner, but in most cases it starts for reasons other than sexual activity, for example after taking antibiotics. Symptoms, including redness and itchiness at the end of the penis, are treated with an antifungal cream. Thrush is more common in women, and a man is unlikely to be the cause of his female partner's thrush. However, if your partner does develop symptoms, it is still worth using an antifungal cream for at least a week, just in case.

Syphilis

Infection with spirochaetes, the spiral-shaped bacteria that cause syphilis, results in the appearance of a painless sore or ulcer (chancre) on the penis, mouth or anus two or three weeks later. The diagnosis is confirmed by examining cells scraped from the surface of this chancre under a microscope. Left untreated, the chancre usually heals up, but the infected individual then enters the second stage of syphilis (which may be a few weeks or a few months later or may even overlap with the first stage), with the development of a fever, headache, rash and enlarged lymph nodes. A blood test will confirm the infection.

Antibiotic treatment, usually an injection of penicillin, eradicates syphilis in most cases. However, regular blood tests are needed over the following two years to make absolutely sure the infection does not recur. If syphilis is not treated in the first or second stage, there is a good chance that the infection will come back many years after the symptoms have disappeared, causing damage to many body organs and tissues, including the heart, aorta, brain and nervous system.

Genital herpes

This STD is caused by a virus, similar to the herpes virus that results in cold sores. An attack of genital herpes characteristically begins with itching or tingling around or on the genitals, followed by the eruption of painful, fluid-filled blisters. These blisters start off clear, turn yellow and then burst, before drying to form scabs that heal slowly.

An initial attack of genital herpes may last up to three weeks; the virus then remains dormant in the genital tissues, causing recurrent symptoms in more than half the men who have been exposed to it. In addition to the painful blistering, there may also be headaches, 'flu symptoms and swollen lymph nodes.

On average, genital herpes will flare up about five times a year, although attacks tend to become less frequent and less severe with age. Treatment with antiviral drugs, such as aciclovir and famciclovir, can speed up healing of the blisters and reduce the number of attacks. A warm salt-water bath can ease the discomfort associated with the blistering, but strong painrelievers may also be required.

To avoid picking up or passing on genital herpes, there should be no sexual contact during an attack. A condom will reduce the risk of spreading this infection during sexual intercourse, but it is not a fail-safe measure.

Genital warts

Genital warts may appear anywhere on the penis or around the anus; they can also grow out of sight inside the urethra or anal canal, in which case the only symptom may be an itch or painless irritation. When they are visible, these warts appear as small bumps or lumps, usually coloured pink or red and growing singly or in clusters. Some are smooth, some are shaped like the outside of a cauliflower.

After someone has been exposed to the human papilloma virus that causes genital warts, the growths may appear at any time over the next few months. They are usually treated by applying the chemical solution podophyllin (available on prescription) to kill the virus and then washing it off a few hours later. Never use any of the ordinary wart-removers from the pharmacist as they are likely to cause pain and irritation. Occasionally, several applications of podophyllin are needed and, if the warts persist, surgical removal may be required.

Once a doctor has checked that the warts have cleared, sexual activity may be resumed. However, genital warts often grow back and need further treatment. Any female partner of a man who has been diagnosed as suffering from genital warts will be advised to have an annual cervical smear because of the proven link between exposure to the wart virus and cervical cancer. A male partner should go to an STD clinic for a check-up as well, even if he does not have any obvious genital warts.

Pubic lice (crabs)

These small, brown, wingless, crab-like creatures, about 2mm long, are usually spread from one person to another during sexual contact, although simply being naked and close to someone with this infection puts you at risk.

Pubic lice latch on to hairs in the genital region and feed off blood by biting the skin. In hairy men, the lice may also be found around the anus. Minute white eggs may be produced by the females and the biting may cause irritation.

Treatment involves application of an insecticide solution (available from the pharmacist) to the infected hairy areas, which is usually left on for up to 24 hours before being washed off. Sexual partners must also be treated and all bed linen should be washed at a temperature of at least 60°C.

Hepatitis B

This potentially fatal liver disease is caused by infection with a virus which can be carried in all body fluids, including semen, saliva, vaginal fluids and blood. Although hepatitis B does not affect the sexual organs, sexual intercourse is one way in which the virus is passed from one person to another. It is also able to survive outside the body for several days in dried blood and on a variety of exposed surfaces. Hepatitis B can be spread by injecting drug users sharing a contaminated needle, as HIV can be, but, unlike HIV, it can also be caught from, for example, an infected toothbrush or razor.

About half of the people who become infected with hepatitis B develop acute inflammation of the liver several weeks or even months later. Symptoms may include loss of appetite, nausea, vomiting, weakness, fatigue, joint pains and jaundice. Many sufferers mistake this illness for an attack of 'flu; others are too ill to do anything but rest in bed, and take months to recover.

Unlike many other STDs, hepatitis B has no cure. Medication may be prescribed to relieve symptoms and to control the effects of any liver damage, but the disease itself has to be allowed to run its own course. In the meantime, the usual advice is to rest in bed, not to drink any alcohol and not take any other drug that has to be processed by the liver.

About 10 per cent of hepatitis B sufferers go on to develop a chronic form of the disease, regardless of the severity of the original infection; even though they don't have any symptoms, these 'silent carriers' can still pass on the disease to others. In addition, many carriers subsequently develop liver cancer, or liver failure due to cirrhosis.

It is not only people with chronic hepatitis B that can spread the infection without knowing about it: the virus can also be passed on even before the initial symptoms have appeared. However, the good news is that there is an effective vaccine to protect against hepatitis B and this is recommended for anyone whose job or lifestyle is likely to put them in contact with the virus, including medical and nursing staff, police and prison warders, homosexuals and heterosexuals with multiple partners, prostitutes, intravenous drug users and any family contacts of these people.

HIV and AIDS

HIV – Human Immunodeficiency Virus – infection may be passed on from one person to another in several different ways:

- by unprotected intercourse (anal or vaginal) with someone who has previously been infected by HIV. If one partner is infected, unprotected anal intercourse carries a particularly high risk of

125

transmitting HIV, but unprotected vaginal intercourse also represents a significant risk

- through inoculation with, or transfusion of, infected blood or blood products. In the UK, since the introduction of improved screening of blood donors and the purifying treatment of plasma products, such as the clotting factor given to haemophiliacs, HIV is unlikely to be passed on in a transfusion. However, infected blood may be injected by a drug user who is sharing contaminated equipment. Also, there have been many cases of dentists, doctors, nurses and laboratory technicians being exposed to HIV when a needle or other instrument has accidentally punctured their skin, although very few have actually become HIV-positive (see below)

- a mother may pass HIV to her baby in the womb, during the delivery, or through breastfeeding.

Although most of the people who have HIV in Britain are homosexuals or injecting drug users (groups recognised as having high-risk behaviour), the fastest-growing group of sufferers have contracted HIV through heterosexual intercourse. It is, however, important to realise that the virus cannot be transmitted simply through casual social contact, for example, touching, cuddling or shaking hands. Nor is HIV passed on by coughing, sneezing, getting an insect bite or from being a blood donor. It is also perfectly safe to share cutlery, crockery, towels and toilet seats.

Symptoms of HIV

This virus invades white blood cells and multiplies inside them. Any time between three weeks and three months after exposure to HIV, symptoms similar to glandular fever (see pages 228–9) may develop, with a high temperature, headache and swollen lymph nodes. These symptoms usually disappear, enabling most people with HIV to continue leading normal lives with no obvious effects on their physical health.

Because HIV results in the formation of specific antibodies to the virus (in which case, the person is referred to as HIV-positive), the diagnosis may be made from a blood test. It takes up to three months for these antibodies to appear, and occasionally as long as six months, so a negative test result is only relevant if that individual has avoided all high-risk activity for at least three months before the test.

Once an adult is confirmed as being HIV-positive, the antibodies won't go away, but he or she may remain in good health for many years.

People who are found to be HIV-positive should take extra care of their health by eating a varied balanced diet, following a regular exercise routine and using relaxation techniques to prevent a build-up of stress. All of these measures will help them stay healthy for longer. They should also take every reasonable precaution to avoid passing HIV on to others.

Drug treatments to slow progression

In 1993, in the UK, the average time for HIV infection to progress to AIDS was eight to ten years. However, with the use of different combinations of anti-retroviral drugs, this time is now expected to increase dramatically.

The anti-retroviral drugs are divided into three main groups: nucleoside analogues, non-nucleoside reverse transcriptase inhibitors and protease inhibitors. They work by reducing the amount of HIV in the body, by stopping the virus replicating itself inside T cells and by stopping newly-produced copies of the virus from infecting more cells.

As a result of reducing the 'viral load' in this way, the damage the virus can cause to the body's immune system is kept under control, and progression of the disease is slowed down.

AIDS and associated illnesses

AIDS – Acquired Immune Deficiency Syndrome – may develop suddenly in someone who has for years been HIV-positive. Sometimes, this progression of the disease is preceded by symptoms such as diarrhoea, weight loss, night sweats and swollen lymph nodes, a phase known as AIDS-related complex.

The onset of AIDS may result in a variety of diseases, most of which are due to the virus causing failure of the body's immune defences against infection and cancer. People with AIDS become more susceptible to infections, such as thrush, shingles, herpes and TB, Kaposi's sarcoma (a rare form of skin cancer) and pneumocystis carinii (an unusual type of pneumonia).

Although the anti-retroviral drugs may slow down the progress of AIDS in most people, they do not provide a cure for HIV and they may also cause serious side-effects. Once AIDS has developed, doctors have to concentrate primarily on treating each complication as it arises, and death is usually due to one of these complications, rather than to HIV.

AIDS and HIV information

The National AIDS Helpline★ provides a free 24-hour service of advice and counselling on HIV and AIDS for all members of the public. The Terrence Higgins Trust★ provides a range of services, including a helpline for people with HIV and AIDS, their families and partners. This charitable organisation can also provide information on self-help groups and other resources which are available in different parts of the UK.

Contraception

There are many different methods of contraception to choose from. With the male contraceptive pill still under investigation, because of the difficulties finding a hormone that is able to suppress sperm development without reducing libido, the male condom remains the only contraceptive currently available for which the man can be directly responsible. However, it is still important for men to be aware of the advantages and disadvantages of other forms of contraception. That way he can be involved in deciding which method would be most suited to both his and his partner's needs, and the mutual support and shared responsibility can only benefit the relationship.

No contraceptive is absolutely fail-safe and all have some disadvantages. It is important to discuss the options in terms of their effectiveness, safety and convenience and to remember the principles of safer sex described earlier; even if the Pill or coil is the woman's first choice of contraceptive in the early stages of a relationship, it is still wise to use a barrier method, such as the male condom, to prevent the possible transmission of STDs such as HIV.

Advice on contraception may be obtained from a GP, family planning clinic or Brook Advisory Centre★ (for young couples aged 25 years or under).

Male condom

The male condom consists of a sheath of thin latex rubber, usually lubricated to make it easier to roll on to the erect penis. Those few men who are allergic to the latex in a condom are usually able to tolerate a special low-allergy brand. Used properly, the male condom is extremely effective, with only two pregnancies per year for every 100 couples relying on this method alone. The number of pregnancies is much higher when the instructions are not followed correctly.

In addition to its contraceptive efficiency, male condoms protect against the transmission of herpes, genital warts, chlamydia and HIV. Men who tend to suffer from premature ejaculation may find that the condom helps by slightly reducing sensory stimulation. The male condom is not suitable for men who often temporarily lose their erection during intercourse, as the condom is likely to slip off.

Because sperm may be present in the lubricating secretions released prior to ejaculation, the condom should always be put on before any genital contact.

Squeezing the tip of the condom while it is being put on prevents air being trapped, which might otherwise increase the risk of it bursting. It is also important not to catch the condom on a fingernail, which might tear it. Before using a condom for the first time, it may be worth practising with one when masturbating to get used to putting it on and taking it off.

After orgasm, but before the erection has completely subsided, your penis should be withdrawn from your partner's vagina. The rim of the condom should be held against your penis to prevent it slipping off and accidentally spilling semen. If penetration lasts longer than ten minutes, it is also a good idea to withdraw to check the condom hasn't been damaged. Never re-use a condom.

A condom may be weakened within seconds of coming into contact with any oil-based lubricant, such as baby oil or Vaseline, so only water-based lubricants, such as KY jelly, should be used. If a massage oil has been used prior to sex, the hands should be wiped before the condom is touched.

Condoms are now on sale in supermarkets, petrol stations and by mail order, as well as in more traditional locations such as pharmacies, barbers and slot machines found in public toilets. Various types of condom – including coloured, ribbed, shaped and flavoured – are available, but only those with a safety kitemark (British Standards Institute or European CE mark) have a guarantee of good quality.

Female condom

This relatively new type of barrier contraceptive consists of a large tube made of very thin polyurethane plastic or rubber with two flexible rings, one at each end, to hold it in place. The ring at the closed end fits inside the vagina while the ring at the open end stays outside, lying flat against the entrance to the vulva and vagina.

During intercourse, you should make sure that your penis passes into the condom and not around it; your partner may need to guide you in during initial penetration. The condom may move during sex, but sperm won't escape into the vagina as long as the penis remains inside the condom. After orgasm, the outer ring of the female condom should be twisted to ensure that the ejaculated semen is retained, then the condom should be gently pulled out.

In addition to protecting against pregnancy, the female condom also helps to prevent the spread of STDs.

Some women are initially put off by the large size of the female condom – it measures over 17×7cm – but these are the actual dimensions of the inside of the vagina. If your partner finds it difficult to fit the female condom at first, she will find it becomes easier with practice. Because it can be put in before intercourse, one advantage is that it does not interrupt love-making. Also, many men find it allows for greater stimulation than the male condom.

Spermicides

Substances which chemically destroy sperm are available as creams, jellies, foams and pessaries. Used on their own, these spermicides are not very effective and if foam or a pessary needs to be inserted into the woman's vagina, this has to be done at least 30 minutes before intercourse to allow it time to dissolve and become active. Some condoms are impregnated with a spermicide to offer additional protection and a spermicide can also be used in combination with a diaphragm or cap for the same reason. There is also evidence to suggest that a spermicide may kill HIV.

Contraceptive sponge

An alternative barrier method of contraception, which uses a spermicide, is the vaginal sponge. This disposable circular polyurethane foam sponge, impregnated with the spermicide nonoxyl-9, is first moistened with water and then pushed high into the woman's vagina before intercourse. One side of the sponge has an indentation that fits over the cervix to form a barrier.

The sponge must be left in place for at least six hours after sex, although it remains effective for up to 24 hours. A loop is attached to the sponge to make it easier to remove, after which it should be thrown away. Even used correctly, the contraceptive sponge is not as effective as either the male or the female condom.

Diaphragm and cap

A diaphragm is a hemispherical dome of thin rubber, with a coiled metal spring inside the rim, which fits diagonally behind the cervix across the front wall of the vagina and extends to the bony ledge at the front of the pelvis. The cervical cap is a smaller, more rigid rubber device which fits snugly over the opening into the uterus by suction.

The family planning doctor will first find the size of diaphragm or cap that fits the woman comfortably. She will then be taught how to insert and remove it herself. A spermicide should be used with the diaphragm or cap to provide additional protection, with extra spermicide inserted into the vagina if intercourse occurs more than once while it is in.

Unlike the sponge, the diaphragm or cap can be used repeatedly. After sex, it should be left in the vagina for at least six hours to prevent any surviving sperm from reaching the uterus.

Oral contraceptive pill

The most commonly prescribed pill contains a combination of synthetic oestrogen and progesterone, which suppress the release of two pituitary gland hormones. As a result, the maturation of eggs inside the ovaries is inhibited and the release of an egg during each menstrual cycle (ovulation) is prevented. In addition to stopping ovulation, the combined pill also thickens the mucus produced by the cervix, making it more hostile to sperm; and it interferes with the development of the uterus lining, which normally happens during the second half of the cycle, to stop implantation, just in case an egg is released and fertilised.

Another type of pill, the so-called mini pill, contains only synthetic progesterone. Although it doesn't always prevent ovulation, its effect on the cervical mucus and uterus lining is normally sufficient to prevent conception. The mini pill is less likely to cause side-effects than the combined pill, but its effectiveness depends on the woman taking it at almost the same time every day, whereas the timing of the combined pill can be less precise.

Your partner may be advised to take the mini pill rather than the combined pill if she is a heavy smoker, is breastfeeding or has a history of high blood pressure, high blood cholesterol, heart disease, migraine, thrombosis or liver disease.

Emergency contraception

If unprotected intercourse with your partner occurs, for example, as a result of a condom splitting or if she has forgotten to put in her diaphragm, it is possible to use an emergency method of contraception sometimes misleadingly referred to as the 'morning after' pill. Your GP or family planning clinic will provide your partner with four tablets, each containing oestrogen and progesterone, two tablets to take immediately and two as a second dose to be taken 12 hours later.

As long as these pills are started within 72 hours of unprotected intercourse, pregnancy can be prevented. Depending on the stage of your partner's menstrual cycle, this relatively high-dose pill will work either by preventing ovulation or by stopping the fertilised egg from implanting.

As another form of emergency contraception, an IUCD (see opposite) can be inserted up to five days after intercourse.

Vaginal ring

This silicone-based rubber ring has a hollow inner core filled with synthetic progesterone. Once inserted high in the vagina, the ring releases small amounts of progesterone continuously, thus having the same contraceptive action as the progesterone-only mini pill (see above).

The advantage of the vaginal ring is that there is no worry over having to take a pill at the same time every day; it is therefore a more reliable contraceptive than the mini pill. Your partner simply has to replace the ring every three months before the supply of progesterone begins to run out.

Intrauterine contraceptive device (IUCD)

An IUCD (coil) is a small plastic device, usually wrapped in thin copper wire, which is inserted inside the uterus by the GP or family planning clinic doctor. The contraceptive effect of an IUCD appears to come from the inflammation it causes inside the uterus, which creates a hostile environment for sperm, as well as making the lining of the uterus unreceptive to implantation of a fertilised egg.

Copper-containing IUCDs can usually be left in the uterus for between three and five years before they have to be replaced. A newer variety of IUCD, which also releases tiny amounts of synthetic progesterone to increase its contraceptive efficiency, has to be changed every 12 months.

Because of the increased risk of pelvic infection, which can lead to infertility, this method of contraception is normally recommended only for older women not planning to have any more children.

Hormone injections

Injections of a long-acting synthetic progesterone can have a reliable contraceptive effect for up to six months. However, this controversial method has generally been reserved for women who cannot cope with other types of contraceptive and has proved unpopular because of the high incidence of side-effects, such as irregular heavy periods and weight gain. Progesterone injections have now been largely superseded by progesterone implants, which first became available in the UK at the end of 1993.

Hormone implants

Six thin, flexible capsules containing synthetic progesterone are inserted, under local anaesthetic, beneath the skin on the inside of the woman's upper arm. Tiny amounts of the progesterone are released continuously into the bloodstream, resulting in the same contraceptive mechanism of action as the progesterone-containing mini pill and vaginal ring.

Clinical trials have shown that hormone implants are at least as effective a contraceptive as the combined pill and more effective than the mini pill and the various barrier methods of contraception. Whereas the progesterone ring has to be changed every three months, the implants remain active for a minimum period of five years. Irregular menstruation is the most common side-effect, but this usually resolves itself within six months.

Natural methods

Natural family planning works on the principle that sexual intercourse takes place only on the days of your partner's menstrual cycle which precede or follow her fertile phase (the rhythm method). However, to determine which days are unsafe it is necessary to predict when ovulation is occurring.

After ovulation, the human egg survives for a maximum of only 24 hours. Sperm are known to be capable of surviving for a maximum of seven days inside one of the fallopian tubes. Therefore, for conception to occur, sexual intercourse must take place within seven days before ovulation, or at some time during the 24 hours after ovulation – the fertile phase of the menstrual cycle.

Unfortunately, prediction of the exact time of ovulation before it occurs is extremely difficult. Although ovulation precedes the first day of menstruation by about 14 days, most women who are not taking the contraceptive pill have variable menstrual cycles, so the actual timing of ovulation may differ from one month to the next by several days. As a result, the safe phase during the first half of the cycle can be highly unpredictable and carries a greater risk of pregnancy than the infertile phase after ovulation.

Your partner can use several techniques to monitor the time at which she ovulates:

- one way is to record her body temperature first thing every morning, before eating, drinking, smoking or taking any exercise, and then to plot these daily readings on a chart. A sudden rise of about 0.5°C occurs at ovulation, a small change but enough to be a reliable predictor as long as the recordings are done correctly using a special fertility thermometer with an easy-to-read scale, and your partner has not for any reason developed a fever. The infertile or safe phase begins on the morning of the third consecutive higher temperature reading
- another sign of ovulation is a change in the cervical mucus, which becomes thicker and less elastic during the second half of the menstrual cycle (i.e. after ovulation)

- the cervix also characteristically feels firmer and moves down a little after ovulation.

To make it more reliable, natural family planning requires proper instruction from an accredited teacher; Fertility UK★ can provide you with a list of teachers in your area. It also demands considerable self-discipline if you are to avoid sexual intercourse on your partner's fertile days. One solution is to use a condom at these times. If you use withdrawal as a contraceptive technique you are highly likely to end up with your partner pregnant, partly because sperm are known to be released in small numbers within the lubricating fluid that appears before ejaculation and also because you may fail to pull your penis clear of the vagina in time.

Sterilisation

Vasectomy

For couples who have decided that they do not want to have any more children, sterilisation of the man by vasectomy is a simple, relatively safe and highly effective procedure. This operation is usually carried out under a local anaesthetic, after which the man can go straight home. Evidence of the popularity of vasectomy comes from the fact that this method of fertility control is now relied on by over half a million couples in the UK.

Considering vasectomy

If you are considering having a vasectomy, you must be as sure as you can be that you have completed your family and will not want any more children under any circumstances. Vasectomy should be regarded as a permanent method of contraception that cannot be reversed.

Before the surgeon agrees to perform a vasectomy, he or she will ensure that someone – usually your GP or a specialist counsellor – has explained the significance of the procedure to you and given you the opportunity to discuss the implications. Ideally, your partner should also be involved in this counselling process, although it is not essential.

It is possible for young men to have a vasectomy, but they are likely to be encouraged to spend longer thinking through their options before confirming their decision. Certainly, any man who admits to going through personal or sexual difficulties at the time he is requesting a vasectomy will be advised against having the operation.

Waiting lists for a vasectomy on the NHS may be several months long in some parts of the UK, although an increasing number of GPs are carrying out this procedure, without charge and with less delay. However long the wait, it is important for couples to continue using some form of reliable contraception in the meantime. A vasectomy done privately will cost about £170–£250, including the consultation, counselling and post-operative sperm counts.

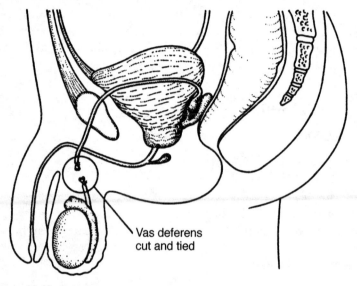

Vas deferens
cut and tied

Figure 10: Vasectomy

The vasectomy operation

Before the operation, any hair on your scrotum will usually be shaved off so that it doesn't get caught up in the stitches. You will probably be asked to shave yourself. After the scrotal skin has been cleaned with antiseptic, a local anaesthetic will be injected under the skin and around each vas deferens (the two tubes that connect each testicle to the urethra). This may cause a slight stinging sensation before the tissues become numb.

Once the anaesthetic has taken effect, one or two small cuts will be made in the skin of the scrotum to reveal the vas deferens. A small piece of each vas deferens is then cut out and the ends either side of the cut bent back and tied with stitches. Throughout this procedure you should not feel any pain, only a pulling sensation (usually in the lower abdomen). To ensure each vas deferens has been correctly identified and cut, the two sections that have been removed may be sent off to the laboratory for examination under a microscope.

Dissolvable stitches are generally used to close the scrotal incision, which is then covered with a sterile dressing. To reduce the amount of discomfort and swelling, you will usually be provided with a scrotal support or advised to wear close-fitting underpants or swimming trunks for a few days. Some men feel faint after a vasectomy, but this sensation usually goes away within 15 minutes.

Recovering from a vasectomy

On the day of the vasectomy, you should go home and take things easy. However, the following day most men are fit enough to return to work as long as their job does not involve strenuous exercise, heavy lifting or driving for long distances. These specific types of activity, and sports that require running or jumping, are best avoided for a week, or at least until the wound discomfort has passed.

Ordinary painrelievers, such as aspirin or paracetamol, should be enough to control any discomfort after a vasectomy, which will usually ease off anyway within a few days. You should wash your scrotum gently in the shower or bath from the day after the operation.

Complications after a vasectomy are extremely rare. There may be some bruising and swelling, but these should disappear within a week or two. Occasionally the wound becomes infected and has to be treated with antibiotics; or a small blood clot forms to cause a painful swelling that has to be removed surgically. The wound itself should have healed completely within ten days and any scar left behind is usually invisible.

Sex after a vasectomy

Sexual intercourse can begin again as soon as the discomfort in your scrotum eases off, but there may be a slight pain associated with ejaculation on the first few occasions. Until all the sperm stored inside the vas deferens have been used up, you are still potentially fertile and must continue with your usual method of contraception until two consecutive semen samples checked in the laboratory have been found to be free of sperm.

The time it takes for all the sperm in each vas deferens to disappear varies between different men, but it usually requires at least ten ejaculations to clear them completely. You will normally be asked to provide a semen sample by masturbation 12 and 14 weeks after the vasectomy and sometimes after a minimum of 20 ejaculations. Further samples will be requested until they become free of any sperm.

Vasectomy should have no effect on orgasm, ejaculation or sexual performance. Semen will continue to be ejaculated. The sperm it would normally contain are still being produced in the testicles but are unable to pass along the vas deferens. They will simply be reabsorbed by the body.

A few men suffer temporary impotence after a vasectomy, which is due to psychological rather than physical factors. This problem usually disappears with reassurance and help from the man's partner to regain his sexual confidence. Occasionally, specialist counselling is needed and if this fails the procedure may have to be reversed.

Long-term complications

The chance of the cut ends of the vas deferens spontaneously rejoining is extremely rare. There have been one or two cases in the past of men getting their partners pregnant several years after a vasectomy, but with modern surgical techniques this is unlikely to happen.

Around half of the men who have had a vasectomy start to produce antibodies against their own sperm. However, this will only be a problem if they request a reversal of the procedure (whereby the cut ends of the vas deferens are rejoined) at a later date, with the aim of having another child.

Female sterilisation

It is estimated that over 1.5 million women in the UK have chosen sterilisation as their method of contraception, having decided they do not want to have any more children. Female sterilisation, like a vasectomy, should be regarded as a permanent method of contraception that cannot be reversed and counselling will therefore be carried out before the operation, ideally with the woman's partner present as well. Some women are able to have their sterilisation reversed at a later date, but there is no guarantee that this will be successful.

Unlike a vasectomy, female sterilisation requires a general anaesthetic and your partner will usually have to remain in hospital overnight. The operation consists of blocking both fallopian tubes to stop eggs from reaching and thus being fertilised by sperm. No further contraception is needed following female sterilisation. Some women experience heavier periods after being sterilised, but it is not known how this is related to the operation as the uterus and ovaries are left as before.

Waiting lists for female sterilisation on the NHS may be as long as two years in some parts of the UK. In the meantime, some other form of contraception should be used. The cost of female sterilisation done privately varies from £475 to as high as £1,200, including the consultation and counselling.

Abortion

Making the decision to have an abortion and then going through with it can be an extremely traumatic experience for a woman. It is also a difficult time for the male partner, who may be experiencing a complex mixture of emotions but is much less likely to be given the opportunity to express his true feelings openly.

Counselling before an abortion can help reduce the emotional impact of terminating the pregnancy and is essential, regardless of whether the reason for the abortion is social, psychological, physical or because of an abnormality in the baby. Even a woman who has definitely made up her mind will find it useful to discuss her feelings with someone who is not emotionally involved with her or her pregnancy.

If your partner is about to have an abortion, it is important for you to show your support by offering to go with her to the doctor or counsellor. You will also benefit from being involved in the discussions. After the abortion, you should be prepared for your partner to go through a variety of emotions, which may include euphoria, anger, guilt, depression and a feeling of numbness, although she may just be relieved that the pregnancy is over. These reactions are perfectly normal, but if symptoms such as depression persist, or become more severe, further counselling and possibly medication may be required.

Making the arrangements

If your partner has decided she doesn't want to continue with her pregnancy, she should see her doctor as soon as possible. The earlier the abortion is performed, the less traumatic it is likely to be both physically and psychologically. Within nine weeks of conception it may be possible for her to be referred for the new abortion pill, avoiding the need for surgery. After 12 weeks it may be more difficult to get an abortion on the NHS in some parts of the UK. Abortions are carried out in NHS hospitals (free of charge) and in charitable or private clinics (where there will be a charge). If your partner doesn't want to be referred by her GP, she can be seen by the local family planning clinic doctor, or she can contact the charitable or private clinic directly.

For a woman to have an abortion, two different doctors must agree that she has reasonable grounds and sign an official form declaring which situation applies in her case. Sometimes the abortion is done because tests have shown the baby has severe abnormalities. However, the usual reason given is that continuing with the pregnancy may threaten the mother's physical or mental health, taking into account social circumstances such as personal relationships, existing children and housing.

Methods of abortion

Whichever technique is used, abortion done under proper medical supervision is a relatively safe procedure, with a low risk of complications, such as infection. Future problems with infertility or miscarriage are no more likely to occur in women who have had a previous abortion.

Abortion pill

Although this relatively new form of medical abortion is licensed to be used in all hospitals and clinics where abortions are carried out, there is a wide variation in the numbers of women offered this procedure in different parts of the UK, depending on the experience and preferences of the medical staff. For example, in Scotland about 50 per cent of early terminations are done by using the abortion pill, compared with an average of 12 to 13 per cent in other regions of the UK. However, it is still worth asking for if the woman's pregnancy is within the nine-week limit.

Initially the woman is given pills which contain mifepristone (RU486), a drug which causes the uterus lining to break down by blocking the action of her progesterone hormones. Vaginal bleeding will usually begin at any time over the next 48 hours. The woman then returns to the hospital or clinic two days later and, if the pills have not already terminated the pregnancy, she will have a pessary containing prostaglandin inserted into her vagina. This pessary will stimulate uterine contractions, which may be painful and accompanied by heavy bleeding, and the termination will be completed within six hours. The woman will then be allowed home, to return for a check-up seven days later.

Vacuum aspiration

The cervix is dilated and a tube is inserted into the uterus and connected to a suction pump to draw out the foetus and placenta. Occasionally, the uterus lining also has to be scraped clear using a sharp spoon-shaped instrument known as a curette.

Prostaglandin infusion

This technique, which may be necessary once a pregnancy passes beyond the 14th week, stimulates the uterus to contract and expel the foetus, rather like inducing labour. Contractions are powerful enough to require painrelievers. The procedure may take up to 24 hours and vaginal bleeding may continue for over a week afterwards.

Trying for a baby

If you and your partner have decided to start a family, you can increase your chance of success by making sure you have intercourse just before the time when your partner is due to ovulate. In contrast to the rhythm method of contraception, described on pages 134–5, in which intercourse is restricted to the infertile phase of the woman's menstrual cycle, the focus of sexual activity is now the fertile phase.

At first, there is no need to worry about predicting the exact time of ovulation. Many couples successfully conceive within a few months by aiming to have sex every other day, particularly during the middle two weeks of the woman's menstrual cycle. However, if this proves unsuccessful, the next stage is to use one of the following techniques to find out when ovulation is occurring.

- If your partner's menstrual cycle is regular, count back 14 days from the day menstruation would be expected to start.

- Your partner should check her temperature each morning using the method described on page 134 to find out when ovulation has taken place. Keeping a temperature chart over several months will generally reveal a consistent pattern and allow ovulation to be predicted before rather than after it actually occurs.
- Your partner may notice that her cervical mucus increases in volume and becomes thinner, clearer and more elastic just before she ovulates, allowing her to stretch an unbroken thread of it between her thumb and forefinger.
- An ovulation-predictor kit can be bought from the pharmacist without a prescription, but these kits tend to be expensive. Your partner can then test her urine, looking for a particular colour change which indicates the presence of a hormone released 24–36 hours prior to ovulation.

Help with conception

A recent survey revealed that only half the couples who had been trying for a baby were successful within the first six months. Another quarter of the couples took a year to conceive and one in five of the remainder had to wait up to two years. You should not, therefore, expect your partner to become pregnant as soon as you stop using contraception. Some delay is normal and does not mean that one or both of you has a problem.

If you have been having unprotected sex regularly (two to three times a week) for over a year without success then you should make an appointment to see a doctor. It is essential that both partners are investigated at the same time because a fertility problem is just as likely to lie with the man as with his partner. Of the estimated one in six couples who are either infertile or having difficulty achieving pregnancy, statistics show that the cause lies with the male in 30 per cent of cases, the female in a further 30 per cent and in the remaining 40 per cent of cases there is either a combination of factors or no cause is ever found.

Some men wrongly assume that if they can get an erection and ejaculate, they are automatically fertile. This is not true, so you should not expect your partner to go through fertility tests on her own. Also, just because you have already fathered children during a previous relationship, for example, doesn't mean you are still fertile.

The doctor is likely to ask all sorts of questions about you and your partner's health and sexual activity, as well as carrying out an examination of your testicles. He or she will want to check that you have been having sex during your partner's fertile phase and will be on the lookout for possible reasons for a fertility problem, such as a history of infection involving the testicles or the presence of a varicocele (varicose vein in the scrotum).

Some of the basic investigations can be done by your GP: for example, sending a sample of your semen to the laboratory for analysis and getting your partner to keep basal body temperature charts for up to six months to check that she is ovulating, and having sex just before ovulation.

Referral to a specialist

Before considering the various tests and treatments for infertility, it is important to be aware of the potential difficulties associated with obtaining the best or most appropriate specialist care. First, although there are NHS hospitals and clinics which offer infertility investigations and treatments, waiting lists tend to be very long and some tests and procedures may not be available. Also, even on the NHS, some charges may be made because of the very high cost of certain treatments.

Some private fertility clinics are subsidised by specialist charities, but it is advisable to check two things before agreeing to receive treatment: the estimated cost and the chance of success. Ask about all the different charges, including the price of repeated cycles of treatment. For example, in vitro fertilisation may cost between £1,500 and £2,200 per cycle, with an extra £300–£500-charge for any additional procedures required (such as PESA, TESE or ICSI – see page 146).

When comparing the success rates of different clinics, it is best to concentrate on the results for couples of similar age groups with similar problems and to ask for the 'take-home baby rates' per cycle of treatment, not just the pregnancy rates. Larger fertility centres tend to have better success rates, but even the best figures are below 30 per cent for some forms of assisted conception.

Information and support

You and your partner should be aware that undergoing tests and treatment for infertility can put a considerable strain on your relationship. It is essential that you support each other through what can be a highly emotional and stressful experience. You should talk honestly about your feelings, be prepared to become angry, frustrated, depressed or anxious at times, but be careful not to start blaming each other for your difficulties.

Fertility clinics generally provide a specially trained counsellor to help couples come to terms with these powerful emotions and to accept the prospect of not being able to have a child of their own. The treatment itself can be extremely demanding, particularly for the woman, and both partners will have to learn to be patient as many months may pass before they are able to move on to the next stage of the process, or to see whether a particular procedure has been successful.

For further information and to be put in contact with a local support group, there are two organisations, ISSUE★ (National Fertility Association) and CHILD,★ run by people who understand the feelings and experiences of couples having difficulty conceiving. In addition, the Human Fertilisation and Embryology Authority★ can provide a list of IVF and artificial insemination centres in the UK.

Causes of male infertility

Scientists have discovered a significant deterioration in the quality of sperm over the last 50 years, the number of sperm in each millilitre of semen having almost halved. There has also been a large increase in the numbers of abnormal sperm and in the proportion of men who have sperm which are less mobile (reduced motility). Environmental pollution is one factor which is being blamed for this decline in male fertility.

However, despite this rather alarming trend, the majority of men are still producing sperm in sufficient numbers and of good enough quality to have no problem with their fertility. Abnormal sperm with excessively large heads, double heads or double tails generally make up less than 20 per cent of the ejaculate, and even when this rises to 50 per cent there should still be enough healthy sperm to achieve conception when everything else is working normally.

The possible causes of male infertility include:

- defects in sperm production, which may be due to a genetic or hormone abnormality, undescended testicles, an environmental factor such as radiation exposure, previous infection like mumps, or an injury

- defects in sperm function, with reduced or absent motility, or inability to penetrate the egg
- obstruction to ejaculation due to an anatomical abnormality, blockage of the vas deferens following an infection like gonorrhoea, or previous vasectomy
- failure of ejaculation, due to impotence, or damage following prostate or other pelvic surgery
- immune system problems, whereby the man or his partner has started to produce antibodies which inactivate or kill his sperm.

Tests for male infertility

In addition to undergoing an examination of the testicles, you will be asked to produce a sample of semen for analysis in the laboratory. You should refrain from ejaculating for about three days before collecting your specimen to provide a sample that represents your best-quality sperm and semen. You will be given a container and, having obtained the sample by masturbating, should deliver it to the laboratory within a few hours, having kept it warm in the meantime.

The sample will be examined under a microscope to check the number of sperm, their shape and how well they move. If any abnormality is found, you will need to provide a second sample, about two weeks later, for a repeat analysis. This is because there can be a considerable natural variation in an individual's sperm count and quality. If, despite following the standard recommendations for improving the production and health of your sperm (see pages 170–2), the abnormality is persistent, you will be referred to a specialist in male infertility (in the UK, usually a urologist).

Additional, more sophisticated sperm tests have been developed over the last few years. These include assessing the ability of sperm to penetrate cervical mucus or to fuse with an egg, and seeing whether chemicals which kill sperm, known as free radicals, are being released in the semen. Other tests to establish the cause of male infertility may include checking the level of a specific hormone in the blood or urine, taking a special X-ray or scan of the testicles to detect a blockage in the vas deferens and, occasionally, examining a biopsy from one of the testicles under a microscope.

One way to see whether your sperm is able to move freely and easily through your partner's cervical mucus is the post-coital test. To do this, you have sex a day or so before ovulation, when the mucus should be at its thinnest and most receptive. Your partner then attends the clinic between 6 and 18 hours later. A sample of mucus is taken from around her cervix to check the survival and fitness of the sperm as they swim through it.

Treatment of male infertility

A few men abstain from sexual intercourse for several weeks at a time in the mistaken belief that this will boost their sperm numbers and quality. In fact, it appears that regular intercourse at three- to four-day intervals gives the best chance of stimulating sperm production.

Treatment of infertility will depend on the specific cause, assuming one can be found. Hormone replacement therapy can help those few men found to have a hormonal abnormality. Surgical re-opening of a vas deferens blocked by scarring due to infection may restore fertility.

Reversal of a vasectomy is often technically successful, but sperm quality may be poor, usually because the vasectomy itself has resulted in the formation of antibodies against the man's own sperm. In men who have started to produce antisperm antibodies, steroid treatment may block this activity and thus enhance their fertility.

For men who have no sperm in their ejaculate, there are now two new techniques in which sperm are collected, either directly from the epididymis – known as Percutaneous Epididymal Sperm Aspiration (PESA) – or directly from the testicles – known as Testicular Sperm Extraction (TESE). Success using PESA or TESE prior to IVF varies depending on the expertise of the medical staff, but in many fertility centres the techniques are as good as IVF itself.

Another new procedure to help overcome male infertility, done in conjunction with IVF, has been designed to counteract the problem of abnormal sperm motility which is thought to be preventing successful penetration of the egg. This technique involves the injection of a single sperm directly into the body of the egg – known as Intracytoplasmic Sperm Injection (ICSI).

Results with ICSI also approach those achieved with IVF in many fertility centres, with a 25 to 35 per cent pregnancy rate per embryo transfer.

Artificial insemination

In this process sperm are injected directly into a woman's cervix. Artificial insemination of a man's own sperm into his partner's cervix may be recommended if the male partner has a persistently reduced sperm count, for example, or where the sperm have difficulty penetrating his partner's cervical mucus. It may also be suggested if a physical disability prevents normal sexual intercourse.

Fresh sperm produced by masturbation are injected within as short a time as possible and the woman remains lying down with the foot of the bed raised for an hour or so afterwards. Insemination is timed to take place just before ovulation and then repeated two to three days later to increase her chance of conception.

Insemination of sperm (kept frozen in a sperm bank) from a donor may be recommended if the man has no sperm, or a sperm count too low for artificial insemination or assisted conception, such as IVF, or if he is known to be a carrier for a particular genetic disease.

Counselling is recommended before donor insemination to make sure the man is completely comfortable about the idea of his partner carrying another man's baby. Although the donor remains anonymous, care is taken to match the male partner's physical characteristics, blood group and, if requested, his religion.

Female infertility

In addition to filling in a basal body temperature chart every day for several months to see whether there is an abrupt rise in mid-cycle that would suggest ovulation is occurring, your partner can undergo various other tests to find possible explanations for her difficulty in becoming pregnant:

- blood tests to identify a hormonal problem that may be interfering with ovulation
- an ultrasound scan to check her ovaries and uterus for disorders such as cysts and fibroids, and to confirm that an egg is being released from one of her ovaries at ovulation
- endometrial biopsy, in which a tiny sample of the woman's uterus lining is removed and examined under a microscope to make sure it is responding to hormonal changes, as well as being free of infection
- laparoscopy, a telescopic examination of her pelvic cavity to check for abnormalities in the shape and position of her uterus, to look for scarring of her fallopian tubes from infection or endometriosis and, by passing a blue dye up through her cervix at the same time, to see whether both fallopian tubes are free of obstruction

147

- X-rays, using a dye which shows up white, to confirm that her fallopian tubes are open.

Treatment of female infertility

If your partner is failing to ovulate each month, she may be prescribed a drug called clomiphene to take by mouth, as well as being injected with a synthetic hormone. Both of these measures stimulate the ovaries to ripen and release one or more eggs. Such drugs must be used extremely carefully to avoid too many eggs being released at the same time.

A blockage or scarring of the fallopian tubes may be corrected by surgical reconstruction, although this is usually successful only when the damage is slight. Women with more severe tubal damage can become pregnant only through an assisted conception technique, such as in vitro fertilisation (IVF).

IVF is not the answer to everyone's fertility problems, but, as well as helping overcome infertility due to blocked or absent fallopian tubes, it can also be successful if your sperm count is persistently low, or if your partner has developed sperm-killing antibodies. Also, there are some couples for whom IVF is successful even though the reason for their infertility has never been found.

To perform IVF, one or more mature eggs are removed from the woman's ovary and then combined outside her body with sperm from either her partner or a donor. The whole procedure is as follows:

- stimulation of ovulation using hormones
- monitoring maturation of the eggs in the ovary, using both ultrasound scanning and blood/urine measurements of the amount of oestrogen these eggs are producing
- injection of a hormone to complete the maturation of the eggs
- removal of the eggs from the ovary through a needle which is guided using ultrasound scanning
- fertilisation of eggs by sperm within a special growth material
- initial development of fertilised eggs in an incubator
- transferring no more than three embryos into the woman's uterus (once they are four to eight cells in size) through a thin tube guided into her cervix; any spares are kept frozen for a later treatment cycle
- pregnancy testing carried out 14 days later, along with an ultrasound scan to check that the tiny embryos have implanted in the uterus.

One large study to determine the percentage of women who achieved a live birth after five IVF cycles produced the following result: 45 per cent for those 34 years old and younger, 29 per cent if they were between 35 and 39, and only 14 per cent for those aged 40 to 45.

Women who need assisted conception but have normal fallopian tubes may be offered an alternative procedure known as gamete intrafallopian transfer (GIFT). The technique is basically the same as IVF, but it is cheaper and easier to perform; the sperm and eggs are kept separate and then transferred one after the other to one of the fallopian tubes, where fertilisation takes place. Any resulting embryo then travels naturally down into the uterus where implantation should occur. GIFT may be recommended if the woman's cervical mucus is hostile to her partner's sperm, or if there is no explanation for the couple's infertility.

Problems with intercourse

If you are suffering from a sexual problem, such as erectile dysfunction (impotence) or premature ejaculation, the first step is to overcome your embarrassment and discuss it with your partner, then, if necessary, seek professional help. The longer you delay visiting the doctor, counsellor or sex therapist, the more likely it is that your sexual difficulties will damage any long-standing relationship in which you are involved. Moreover, left untreated, sexual problems may cause depression or a build-up of anxiety, which will only make matters worse.

Your own GP may be one of the increasing number of doctors who have undertaken additional training in psychosexual therapy, and may therefore be able to offer help. Specialist sex therapy and counselling for sexual problems are also available on the NHS, but this service is very restricted in some parts of the UK and waiting lists are weeks, even months, long.

If you can afford to pay for private therapy, you could ask your GP to recommend a specialist, or you could contact Relate★ (formerly the Marriage Guidance Council) or the British Association for Sexual and Marital Therapy★ for details of suitable sex therapists in your area. A number of good books are available, too, on the subject of sexual difficulties and how to overcome them.

The following section explains the possible causes of the most common psychosexual problems in men and gives some simple advice on self-help measures, as well as information on the sort of therapy that a specialist might recommend.

Reduced sex drive

Most men lose interest in sex at some time. This becomes a problem only if nearly every time your partner wants sex, you do not. Many different factors can reduce the sex drive (libido); the first step towards restoring an interest and appetite for sex is therefore to try to identify the most likely reasons.

Stress commonly reduces libido, particularly money worries, overwork, or fear of losing your job. Fatigue is another common reason, as is anxiety or depression. If you feel under stress, a regular relaxation exercise (see Chapter 3) and adjustment of your lifestyle will boost your emotional health, as well as your sex drive. When anxiety or depression is severe enough to interfere with your ability to live a normal life, including making love, it is time to ask your GP for help.

Not surprisingly, physical illnesses can also reduce libido, but, assuming the disease can be treated, an interest in sex should return as part of the recovery. Various drugs, such as blood pressure medication or sleeping tablets, can also lower the drive; your doctor should be able to suggest alternative medication.

Boredom may be a problem. The easy answer here, and the one that explains why so many marriages and partnerships break up every day, is to look for sexual excitement elsewhere. However, assuming you do want your relationship to work, there is much you can do to put the sparkle back in your sex life at home. For example, you should:

- talk to your partner about his or her sexual needs
- spend time stimulating your partner (and *vice versa*) before moving on to actual intercourse
- enjoy sex, not just the orgasm
- address any problems you and your partner are having outside the bedroom
- consider counselling if you and your partner are unable to talk over your difficulties yourselves.

Erectile dysfunction (impotence)

Erectile dysfunction, usually referred to as impotence, has received phenomenal media attention since the launch in 1998 of new treatments such as Viagra. Although virtually all men will experience impotence at some time in their lives, it is usually only as a temporary reaction to either stress, anxiety, fatigue or drinking too much alcohol. However, if we use the stricter definition of impotence – being consistently unable to get an erection or maintain an erection during sexual intercourse – about three million men are believed to suffer from this problem in the UK.

Many men with erectile dysfunction mistakenly believe that it must be the result of a psychological problem, such as being overstressed – a belief that may keep them from seeking medical treatment. Although psychological factors can play a role for some men, and impotence will almost inevitably have a psychological effect on the man, most cases of erectile dysfunction are associated with physical conditions or their medication, such as:

- disorders that affect the blood vessels and restrict blood flow to the penis, such as diabetes, heart disease, high blood pressure or high cholesterol
- conditions that interrupt the normal connection between the central nervous system and the penis, such as prostate surgery, traumatic injury, multiple sclerosis or Parkinson's disease
- depression (see page 216–18)
- medications (including some used to treat high blood pressure and depression) that bring about impotence as an unwanted side-effect.

Some men wrongly assume that erection problems are a natural consequence of ageing. It is true that as a man grows older, he can expect some changes in his sex life, for example it may take him a bit longer to get aroused or he may require more intense or prolonged stimulation to achieve a satisfactory erection. It is also true that erectile dysfunction is more common among older men because they are more likely to have conditions that can cause impotence, such as heart disease or diabetes, and they are more likely to be taking medications that may impair erectile function. However, regardless of his age, a man should seek medical help for impotence if he wants to remain sexually active.

Embarrassment is another reason why a lot of men avoid seeking help for impotence. As with other medical conditions, many men with impotence are reluctant to see their GP and are even more reluctant to discuss their problem openly with their partner. As a result, this can put a terrible strain on relationships and can often lead to a couple splitting up. The man may start to avoid sexual contact or physical intimacy, fearing that he will not be able to 'perform'. His partner may wrongly assume that he is no longer attracted to her or him, or that he is having an affair with someone else.

ERECTIONS AND WHAT CAN GO WRONG

Without sexual stimulation only a limited amount of blood flows into the penis, keeping it flaccid (soft, i.e. not erect). When a man is sexually aroused, the arteries in the penis relax and widen to allow more blood to flow into it. In fact, the erect penis contains roughly seven to eight times more blood than when it is flaccid. As the penis expands, the veins that normally carry blood away from the penis become compressed, which in turn restricts how much blood can flow out of the penis. With more blood flowing in and less flowing out, the penis enlarges to become erect.

If the blood vessels or nerves associated with this process are not working properly, due to, for example, damage from diabetes, a man may no longer be able to get an erection. The problem often lies with the small blood vessels leading out of the penis, which lose their ability to constrict and trap blood within the spongy tissues known as the corpora cavernosa. It is the trapped blood that gives the erect penis its rigidity.

First steps to solving the problem

Although most cases of impotence are due to a physical disorder, it is still important to consider first whether it might actually be the result of a problem in your relationship. If you are having relationship difficulties that you are unable to sort out yourselves, then your doctor can refer you for counselling or to a sex therapist depending on the nature of the problem.

Erectile dysfunction may also be overcome simply by discussing with your partner ways to vary your lovemaking, explaining what extra stimulation might help you achieve and maintain your erection. Oral sex is particularly effective at getting the blood flowing into the penis. If prolonged stress is the underlying cause of your impotence, taking steps to reduce stress overload will usually help you relax enough to enjoy your sex life again.

Some men can help restore their erectile function by starting a routine of pelvic-floor muscle exercises, the same type of exercise that women follow after childbirth to restore their vaginal tone and regain control of their urinary stream. To do this simple exercise, try stopping and starting in mid-flow when you pass urine. Begin by stopping the flow for a count of four seconds and focus on the muscles you use, then contract the same muscles again for at least four seconds when you have finished. After one week, try contracting the muscles for a longer count of up to eight to ten seconds. You should notice an improvement in your erections within four to twelve weeks.

Various prescription drugs, including certain blood pressure treatments, antihistamines, sedatives and antidepressants, can cause impotence as one of their side-effects. In such cases, you should check with your doctor to see whether switching to an alternative drug could help you. Smoking may increase the risk of impotence, as might alcohol abuse or any type of recreational drug. Men who are overweight may boost their sexual performance by shedding a few kilograms, which may also improve their self-image and their self-confidence.

An abnormally low testosterone level is thought to be the cause of impotence in only about two to three per cent of cases, most of whom are men over the age of 65 (see also 'Male menopause', pages 166–8). In these few cases, hormone replacement therapy, with testosterone administered in the form of an implant under the skin, or a skin patch, will usually be prescribed only if tests have confirmed a deficiency of this sex hormone. Also, testosterone cannot be given to men who have a previous history of prostate cancer, heart or liver disease

What about Viagra?

Sildenafil citrate (Viagra) has been hailed as the new 'wonder drug' for impotence. Launched in September 1998 in the UK, Viagra – available on prescription – can improve a man's natural response to sexual stimulation by increasing the blood flow to his penis.

In clinical studies, Viagra improved erections in about three out of four men, compared with only one out of four who received placebo (pills that look like the drug being tested but do not contain the active ingredient). Men in these trials also reported that with Viagra two out of three attempts resulted in successful sexual intercourse (compared with only one out of five attempts for patients on placebo).

About one hour before engaging in sexual activity, the man takes one Viagra tablet and, within about 30 minutes (longer if he has just eaten a fatty meal) and for up to 4 hours afterwards, it can help him get an erection in response to sexual stimulation. However, he will not get an erection just by taking the pill; in other words unless he is sexually stimulated, Viagra will not give him an erection. Viagra is neither a sex hormone nor an aphrodisiac, it simply improves the erectile function of a man who has impotence, by increasing blood flow to his penis while he is sexually aroused.

As with all prescription medicines, it is important to discuss with your doctor whether Viagra is suitable for you. For example, Viagra should never be taken by any man who is also taking a class of drugs known as nitrates (such as glyceryl trinitrate, commonly prescribed to treat angina), as in combination these drugs can lower blood pressure to dangerous levels.

Some men experience side-effects with Viagra, including headaches, facial flushing, upset stomach and occasionally a visual disturbance, where images become blurred or tinged with a blue colour. These side-effects are generally mild, go away in a short time and do not cause patients to stop taking Viagra. To reduce the risk of complications, it is important not to take Viagra more often than once a day.

Although many thousands of men have already benefitted from Viagra, a few who have taken it have died as a result of a heart attack, which is why men with a heart condition are advised against taking this drug without first discussing the risks with their doctor.

What about MUSE?

Another new treatment for impotence, which has been found to be effective, involves the insertion of the drug alprostadil (a synthetic prostaglandin), in the form of a pellet the size of a small grain of rice, through the urethral opening at the tip of the penis. This transurethral technique, known as MUSE, uses a special disposable device that automatically releases the pellet when a button on the applicator is depressed.

MUSE works by relaxing the muscles within the erectile tissue of the penis to cause an erection within five to ten minutes. The procedure can be used twice within 24 hours, but leaving at least one hour between the first and second occasion.

In one study, 65 per cent of the men treated with MUSE achieved an erection sufficient for intercourse, compared with only 19 per cent who were given placebo (inactive) pellets to insert. However, one third of the men given a pellet of alprostadil failed to produce an erection.

The number of men reporting that they were able to have sex over the ensuing three months using MUSE was three and a half times higher than in the placebo group. In addition, 64 per cent of the MUSE patients reported having at least one orgasm, compared with only 24 per cent of the placebo recipients.

To increase the chance of success with MUSE, proper instruction from the clinic nurse is essential, in addition to using the accompanying patient information leaflet and/or training video.

One drawback is that MUSE can cause some discomfort on insertion, but this is not usually bad enough to stop most men continuing with it. The discomfort can be reduced, and the absorption of the drug speeded up, if the urethra is moist prior to insertion of the pellet – the man is therefore advised to pass urine first and then gently shake his penis to remove drops of urine. The other disadvantage is that because alprostadil passes from the man's circulation into his semen and may damage a developing foetus, condoms should be used during sexual intercourse if the man's partner is or may become pregnant.

What about vacuum therapy?

Another effective method of dealing with impotence, which is painless and relatively easy to use, is vacuum therapy. This method, which has been used successfully by several thousand men in the UK since the mid-1980s, produces an erection prior to intercourse using a cylinder attached to a hand- or battery-driven pump.

Having liberally applied lubricant to the open end of the cylinder, the man places his penis inside and then creates a partial vacuum around it by pumping out the air. As a result, blood is drawn into the penis and it becomes erect within minutes. A constriction band is then slipped from around the cylinder on to the base of the penis to maintain the erection.

Reported success rates with vacuum therapy vary from 60 to 90 per cent, and this technique seems to be particularly useful for diabetics who have nerve and blood vessel damage as a result of their condition. The band can be left on safely for up to 30 minutes and, as soon as it is removed, the erection will go.

To increase the chance of success with vacuum therapy, proper instruction is essential from the accompanying booklet and/or video, as well as patience, practice and, above all, a supportive partner.

Occasionally, vacuum therapy may cause bruising, particularly if the air is drawn out too quickly or the constriction band is left on too long. Also, the man may need to trim his pubic hair to avoid it getting trapped in the cylinder. Other disadvantages are that the penis will feel cold to touch and that the erection will hinge from where the ring has been positioned, rather than from the true base of the penis within the lower abdomen. This means that although the penis should be stiff enough for intercourse, the couple may need to find different sexual positions for intercourse to be comfortable.

The cost of a vacuum pump and accessories may vary from £150 to £320, depending on the model selected. They are not generally available on the NHS, although a few clinics will lend out pumps.

What about injection therapy?

Another treatment for impotence, especially useful in men who do not respond to the other methods, involves self-injection of either the prostaglandin alprostadil (Caverject, Viridal) or the selective alpha-1-blocker moxisylyte (Erecnos) into the shaft of the penis using a very fine needle. Pressure then has to be applied to the injection site for two to three minutes to prevent bleeding.

Injection of one of these drugs usually produces a good enough erection for intercourse within 10 to 15 minutes, which lasts for up to 30 to 60 minutes. It works by dilating the blood vessels inside the penis, even in men whose blood vessels have been damaged by diabetes.

In addition to pain from the injection, and occasionally tender scarring at the injection site, some men develop a condition known as priapism, in which the erection persists for several hours and becomes painful. The erection may subside with exercise but, if it does not, the man will need an injection of an adrenaline-like substance to return the penis to a flaccid state and prevent permanent damage to the erectile tissues.

Nowadays, self-injection treatment is available on the NHS. Although very few NHS impotence clinics exist, you can ask your GP to prescribe the injection treatment and, if he or she is unable to instruct you on how to inject yourself, you may be referred to to a urology clinic. In addition, in some parts of the UK, there are specialist impotence clinics for diabetics, which are also prepared to see other men as well.

Will my GP be supportive?

GPs differ widely in their knowledge and experience in the management of erectile dysfunction. While a few operate their own specialist impotence clinics, unfortunately many can be quite dismissive of this condition. However, you should not hesitate to ask to be referred to an NHS clinic – the Impotence Association* can provide you with a list of clinics in your part of the UK.

The cost of a private consultation combined with the drug charges can add up to several hundred pounds for a treatment you could be getting free but, if you are going to have to wait a long time for instruction at an NHS clinic, you could be seen privately and then, to save money, get your supplies from your GP.

What about penile implants?

When impotence cannot be satisfactorily reversed by any of the above methods, the only solution may be surgical insertion of an artificial penile implant. Following a period of hospitalisation after surgery, it will be six to eight weeks before the man is able to have sexual intercourse again.

Although these implants are an effective way of achieving an erection, they should be regarded as a last resort, as surgery irreversibly destroys normal erectile tissue and, occasionally, the implant becomes infected or damaged and has to be removed.

The simplest form of penile implant consists of two semi-rigid rods with a silicone coating. Following surgery, the penis can be bent upwards for sexual intercourse and pointed downwards to conceal the erection at other times. However, the size of the penis will not alter during intercourse. Another disadvantage is that this type of implant is difficult to conceal under swimming trunks or tight clothing.

Alternatively, you can use a hydraulic device, which can increase the girth of the penis. Cylinders are implanted inside the penis and connected to a pump in the scrotum and a reservoir of fluid under the abdominal muscles. Squeezing the pump forces fluid from the reservoir into the cylinders to produce an erection; a release valve can be activated to return the fluid to the reservoir after intercourse, leaving the penis flaccid once again. The latest version is totally self-contained within the penis.

Pain during intercourse

Although dyspareunia (painful intercourse) is much less common in men than women, there are several medical disorders which can cause pain or discomfort for a man during sexual intercourse. If symptoms are interfering with your love life, you should make an appointment to see a doctor.

Possible causes of dyspareunia in men, all of which can be treated to relieve the discomfort, include balanitis (inflammation of the glans of the penis usually due to infection, but sometimes the result of an allergy to a spermicide or condom), phimosis (a tight foreskin) and Peyronie's disease (deformity of the penis due to scar tissue). These penis disorders are all discussed in more detail in Chapter 6. Inflammation of the prostate gland may sometimes cause stabbing pains at the tip of the penis, particularly during sexual intercourse.

Premature ejaculation

Occasional episodes of premature ejaculation, in which the man ejaculates almost immediately on, or even before penetration, occur in most men at some time in their love life. If you are anxious, the risk of your ejaculating prematurely increases, which is why it is more likely to happen when you are first having sex with a new partner. Unfortunately, even the worry that you might ejaculate before you have satisfied your partner is often enough to cause this common sexual problem.

The method usually recommended by sex therapists to help a man gain more control over ejaculation is the 'squeeze technique'. He asks his partner to firmly squeeze the head of his penis between her or his thumb and forefinger for a count of 10 each time he feels the urge to ejaculate. This squeeze, which should not hurt, reduces the desire to ejaculate, allowing further stimulation to continue.

After practising the squeeze technique a few times during masturbation, you can try penetrative intercourse, withdrawing to have the penis squeezed each time you experience the sensations of impending ejaculation, until you feel ready to ejaculate. With patience and the co-operation of your partner, you should soon learn to hold back from ejaculating, without needing to stop for a squeeze.

Delayed ejaculation

Ejaculation in men occurs as a reflex response to continued stimulation of the erect penis. Occasionally, ejaculation does not happen, regardless of how long sexual intercourse continues, a condition known as delayed ejaculation. For most men, an isolated episode of delayed ejaculation has a simple explanation – they may have drunk too much alcohol, may be tired, may find a particular brand of condom is making intercourse less stimulating, or may already have ejaculated recently.

If you suffer from delayed ejaculation as a recurrent or continuous problem, you may have some underlying anxiety, of which you are not aware, about ejaculating into your partner . This may be related to a strict upbringing, hostile feelings towards your partner, or even the fear of a female partner becoming pregnant. To resolve these deep-rooted emotions, you and your partner may need counselling from a specially trained therapist.

The method usually recommended by sex therapists to help someone overcome the problem of delayed ejaculation is for a man to have intercourse until his partner is satisfied, then to withdraw his penis so that stimulation can be continued by masturbation. When the sensation of impending ejaculation is experienced, penetration is resumed so that ejaculation into his partner is inevitable. With the co-operation of their partners, most men find that after ejaculating during penetration on several occasions they start to find this much easier to do, without needing to stop for additional manual stimulation.

Homosexuality

Alfred C. Kinsey, an American sex expert, carried out a survey among over 4,000 white American adult men in the late 1940s which revealed that about four per cent were exclusively homosexual. A similar incidence of male homosexuality has been found in subsequent surveys conducted in the UK and continental Europe, as well as in the USA. However, a 1993 UK survey by Kaye Wellings *et al* has suggested that of nearly 19,000 people interviewed in the early

1990s the incidence of exclusive homosexuality in men was much lower – closer to one per cent.

Homosexual encounters are common in adolescent boys coming to terms with their sexuality. They are generally regarded as a normal part of sexual development and are certainly nothing to feel guilty or upset about. In their teens, boys tend to develop intense relationships with other boys, regardless of whether they are in a mixed school or not. This bonding may include physical attraction and can lead to sexual contact, usually in the form of mutual masturbation.

The proportion of men who have experienced some form of homosexual activity at some stage in their life is thought to be about one in ten. Predictably, this figure is even higher in an environment such as a prison, where men are forced to live together without heterosexual contact. Homosexual relationships under these circumstances fulfil the need for an emotional outlet as well as relieving sexual tension. However, heterosexuals usually return to heterosexual activity as soon as the opportunity arises again.

Men who remain sexually attracted to both men and women all their lives, and whose erotic fantasies are almost equally divided between men and women, are in fact in a tiny minority. Men who appear to be bisexual because they are married or living with a female partner are in fact invariably homosexual – they may have married or moved in with a female partner before they discovered they were gay. Also, a number of men persevere with a heterosexual relationship in an attempt to deny their homosexuality, to disguise it from others or in response to pressure to conform socially.

A heterosexual relationship may continue because of the love and affection the homosexual man feels for his female partner, even if that love is not satisfying his physical and erotic desires. However, it may be best for the man to 'come out' to his female partner, regardless of the original motivation behind their relationship, out of respect for her as well as for the selfish reason of assisting the development of his own sexual identity. When and how he goes about revealing his homosexuality depends very much on his individual circumstances.

Finally, it is important to distinguish between the desire for physical contact with other men and contact which has sexual connotations. Many men hold back from touching or hugging another man because they worry that this will be misinterpreted as latent homosexuality.

Defining homosexuality

Male homosexuality is more than just a physical attraction to another man. Broadly speaking, it is a preference for emotional and physical contact with men rather than women, for example when a man responds erotically to other men or has sexual fantasies about other men. It does not necessarily include any sexual activity with men.

Whatever fixed images and stereotypes the media may try to put across, homosexuals are as highly individual in their sexuality and relationships as are heterosexuals. Only a few display 'camp', overtly feminine behaviour and mannerisms.

Homosexual relationships do not necessarily involve anal intercourse (legal in the UK only between consenting males over the age of 18). There are many other ways in which two men can give each other sexual pleasure. While it is true that homosexual men are more likely than heterosexuals to have random, casual sexual encounters, this is not characteristic of all homosexual males. It is also important to remember that promiscuity is common among heterosexual males.

'Coming out'

For some young men, homosexual feelings and attractions are not just a phase they are going through as part of their sexual development. Realisation of their homosexuality will usually occur at some time between the ages of 8 and 14. While many homosexual men are unable to remember their first same-sex erotic impulses or fantasies, they often recall certain behavioural characteristics which set them apart from their peers: for example, they may have avoided aggressive play or felt themselves to be more sensitive than other boys.

It can be extremely difficult for a young man to acknowledge his homosexuality. Even though it is becoming increasingly accepted as an alternative lifestyle, with society's attitudes steadily more liberal over the past 20 years, there is still a great deal of hostility, intolerance and discrimination towards and oppression of homosexual men. A homosexual adolescent may try to deny his sexuality initially because of fears of persecution, teasing or bullying, for example. Later in life, he may be worried about it affecting his chances of getting a job.

Unfair treatment of homosexual men has been made worse by the AIDS epidemic (see pages 118–19 and 125–8), homosexuals having been falsely accused of being solely responsible for the existence and

161

spread of the infection. Other common myths which encourage homophobic attitudes are that homosexual men are sexually aggressive or that they are more likely to molest children.

With all this prejudice, it is not surprising that homosexual men sometimes try to suppress their true sexuality. Rather than making their lives easier, however, this denial leads to greater stress and unhappiness. Only when a homosexual man has learnt to love and respect himself as a homosexual can he go on to develop his sexual identity and form satisfactory relationships with other men. Continued denial is likely to lead to depression, isolation, alienation and a progressive erosion of self-esteem.

Often, an important step towards coming to terms with his homosexuality is for a man to 'come out' to his parents. They may initially be upset by the news, but this reaction may reflect their concern for his future happiness and well-being, rather than being a sign that they don't unconditionally love their son. In some cases, rather than confronting his parents with his homosexuality, he may simply prefer not to disguise the fact, to allow them to come to terms with it in their own way.

Although coming out is a highly individual experience, it can be facilitated by involvement in gay social networks. These make it easier to form non-sexual and sexual relationships with other gay men. For some men, confusion about their true sexuality can last for several years, but they can be reassured that there is no need to decide immediately where their preferences lie.

Explaining male homosexuality

Some doctors and psychologists try to explain away homosexuality as a pathological condition which, once the cause has been identified, can be treated and even 'cured'. For example, there have been some attempts to explain homosexuality in terms of emotional conditioning and a particular type of parenting during childhood.

Much has been written about the influence of specific parent models in determining the subsequent sexuality of a male child. It has been suggested that a powerful mother who has an intense relationship with her son can undermine his masculinity and inhibit the development of his sexual independence, and that a weak, detached or non-existent relationship with his father will make it even more difficult for the son to separate emotionally from his domineering mother. However, most homosexual men come from a normal home environment and, besides, unsatisfactory parental relationships also apply to large numbers of heterosexual men. In reality, such disruption of emotional development during childhood or adolescence is more likely to affect a man's ability to form sexual relationships of any kind, than to influence his sexual orientation.

In the past, psychologists have even tried to use aversion therapy to convert a homosexual into a heterosexual man. It was thought that by giving an electric shock to a man each time he responded to an erotic picture of a male (but not when pictures of females were shown), he would learn to associate male erotica with pain and change his sexual preference as a result. Not surprisingly, aversion therapy failed to work in the long term and also risked seriously damaging the self-image of the man, by reinforcing the perception that society regards homosexuality as undesirable.

Biological differences

The possibility of there being a biological difference between heterosexual and homosexual men has been the subject of a considerable amount of research. No evidence has been found, however, of any significant differences in the levels of the male sex hormone testosterone.

A study published in the American journal *Science* (30 August 1991) reported that a comparison of brain samples taken from heterosexual and homosexual men who died of AIDS showed a significant difference in the average size of a particular cell structure (INAH 3) inside the hypothalamus – the gland at the base of the brain which is associated with emotional response. The author of the study, Le Vay of the Salk Institute in Southern California, has argued that this difference is the result of hormonal action while the baby is developing inside his mother's womb. However, it may be that these changes are a consequence rather than a cause of an individual's sexual orientation. Also, other factors may influence this structure.

Finally, there has been a tremendous amount of publicity surrounding the possible existence of a 'gay gene'. Also in *Science* (16 July 1993), an American team of scientists reported the discovery of genetic markers on the tip of the X-chromosome – the sex chromosome inherited from the mother – which appear to be strongly linked to being homosexual. This study (carried out by Dr Dean

Hamer and colleagues at the National Cancer Institute in Washington) was based on a detailed examination of the genetic make-up of over 100 homosexual men and their family trees. It is now hoped that the exact gene or genes which predispose a man to homosexuality can be identified.

The concept of a genetic basis to homosexuality continues to be heavily criticised in some quarters. If there does turn out to be a gay gene, this should only further emphasise that homosexuality in a man is as much a part of his persona as the colour of his hair or eyes, not a disorder that needs treatment.

Sexual deviation

Sexual deviation is any form of behaviour or activity that goes beyond what is regarded as socially acceptable and can be any of a variety of sexual practices which in no way enhance the love and affection that individuals feel for one another within a relationship. Most men who experience deviant sexual urges are uncertain of their masculinity; many, having failed to form any normal fulfilling sexual relationship with women or other men, feel sexually inadequate as a result. There also seems to be a tendency for adults who were sexually abused as children either to begin sexually deviant behaviour that involves abuse of others, or to continue being victims of abuse in adulthood.

Examples of sexual deviation include:

- voyeurism, whereby arousal is achieved by secretly watching other people have sex or get undressed, often accompanied by masturbation
- exhibitionism, in which exposure of the genitals to unsuspecting women causes sexual excitement, again often accompanied by masturbation, although only rarely associated with violence towards a victim
- transvestism, which means dressing in the clothes of the opposite sex to gain pleasure and often sexual excitement
- frottage, whereby a man becomes aroused by rubbing his genitals against a woman's body while pushed together in a crowd
- urophilia (or coprophilia), in which sexual excitement is a response to being urinated on (or defecated on)
- bestiality, which is sexual activity or intercourse with an animal

- sadism (or masochism), in which sexual arousal results from the infliction of pain or violence towards (or from) someone
- fetishism, which becomes deviant behaviour when an individual experiences more sexual excitement with the fetish (object) than with its owner
- paedophilia, which is sexual activity or intercourse with a child.

Men who are prepared to seek treatment to control sexually deviant behaviour may respond well to psychosexual counselling, psychotherapy, or therapy from a psychologist which focuses on substituting alternative patterns of sexual behaviour that are socially acceptable. A GP should be able to recommend a suitable therapist without making any moral judgement about the sexual urges or fantasies described.

Sexual identity problems

One man in every 30,000 desperately wants to change his male sexual characteristics for those of a female, and to live his life as a woman. Transsexualism has nothing to do with homosexuality (sexual attraction to people of the same sex) or with transvestism (see above). A transsexual man feels he was born into the wrong body, and will want to dress as a woman, permanently and as a natural response to his desire to become a female.

Research into the cause of transsexualism suggests that sexual identity is determined primarily by the way a man was treated by his parents when he was a child. If a boy's parents subconsciously or consciously wanted a girl, then there is a greater chance that he will grow up unhappy with his sexual identity than if his parents had consistently treated him as a boy. This emotional conditioning is obviously a powerful phenomenon as it can override the genetic and hormonal factors that normally determine male sexual identity.

Before a transsexual man is considered for sex-change surgery, he will usually have to demonstrate that he has been successfully living as a woman for at least two years. A psychiatrist will check there is no significant mental disorder, such as schizophrenia. The man will then be referred to a gender reassignment programme, which includes counselling on dress and behaviour, as well as initiation of female sex hormone therapy.

Sex-change surgery is not just physically traumatic, bringing permanent infertility and impotence, it can also cause considerable psychological and psychosexual trauma. However, by carefully integrating the man into his new sexual role, the risk of serious emotional disturbance can be reduced and many transsexuals find peace of mind for the first time in their lives once the transformation has been achieved.

Male menopause

Middle-aged men often complain of a variety of symptoms similar to those suffered by women going through the menopause. Men may not suffer from hot flushes and night sweats, but they certainly can experience many of the others, such as headaches, loss of memory, difficulty making decisions, lack of confidence, lethargy, exhaustion and depression. In contrast to menopausal women, men can retain their fertility well into old age; however, surveys show that middle-aged men notice a steady decline in their sex drive and are more likely to have difficulties getting and maintaining an erection, as a result of which their sexual performance can suffer.

Currently medical experts disagree as to whether this common phenomenon among men, popularly referred to as the mid-life crisis, is hormonal (like the female menopause) or purely psychological. The menopause in women is associated with a dramatic reduction in the production of the female sex hormone, oestrogen, by the ovaries. In men, there is a drop in the production of the male sex hormone, testosterone, by the testicles; but this tends to be only a gradual reduction and it usually starts much later in life, after the age of 60.

One possible explanation for the symptoms of male menopause in men in their 40s and 50s is that some factor stops testosterone working normally – even though the absolute level of testosterone may still be normal.

Testosterone replacement therapy

Clinical research has suggested that testosterone therapy may sometimes be effective at relieving symptoms of the male menopause, or viropause, as it has become known. About 1,000 men between the ages of 30 and 80 received treatment with testosterone at one private clinic in London and a moderate to marked improvement was reported in more than 80 per cent.

Testosterone is initially prescribed in tablet or capsule form for the first few months. If this treatment is successful, pellets of testosterone may then be implanted into the buttock to produce a long-term benefit, lasting up to six months.

The testosterone skin patch has also been used as an alternative to an implant, but may cause redness and blistering of the skin as a side-effect. Men who receive testosterone therapy have a thorough health check first and, because of the possible link between testosterone treatment and prostate cancer, various screening tests are carried out to exclude this particular disease.

However, until carefully controlled clinical trials are organised to confirm the true benefits of testosterone, male hormone replacement therapy is likely to remain highly controversial. Treatment can only be obtained privately and the bill, for screening tests, drugs and consultations, is likely to add up to several hundred pounds.

Psychological factors

The female menopause is universally accepted as being the result of oestrogen deficiency, but it is also recognised that various psychological factors may contribute to the symptoms. In middle-aged men, the mid-life crisis is thought by most doctors in the UK to be purely a reaction to stress and other emotional pressures, with no relationship to testosterone deficiency.

There is no easy answer for those trying to negotiate a smooth passage through middle age. However, there are a few measures that can protect your emotional health and help to sustain any long-term relationship you are in:

- take positive steps to prevent stress overload at work and at home
- follow a regular exercise routine to help you stay in good physical shape
- work hard at keeping the romance and sparkle in your relationship; if you are having sexual difficulties with your partner, try to talk openly about them and do not put off seeking professional help
- make the effort to get involved in new challenges, both physical and intellectual
- try not to resent your partner if he or she is developing a new role or career, or seems to be more successful than you are.

Genital cosmetic surgery

For those few men whose penis is short enough to prevent them enjoying a normal sex life, there is a plastic surgery procedure which involves cutting through the suspensory ligament across the top of their penis where it passes into the lower part of the abdomen. However, even though this operation can give more length to the penis, it also makes it more unstable during sexual intercourse.

In a desire to make the base of their penis wider, some men undergo a penis-enlarging operation, called circumferential autologous penile engorgement (CAPE). This procedure involves the removal of about 30ml of fat from the centre of the abdominal wall through a suction tube; this fat is then injected in several different areas around the shaft of the penis, just underneath the skin.

As a result, the penis becomes more bulky, with an increase in circumference of several centimetres. Not only does the man get to show a bigger bulge in his swimming trunks, but by having the base of his penis widened it is claimed that he will be able to achieve greater stimulation of the nerve endings in the outer part of a woman's vagina during penetrative intercourse.

Although over 1,000 American males have undergone this operation, which is done under local anaesthetic, takes up to an hour to perform and costs the equivalent of over £2,000, it has only rarely been carried out in the UK. One problem is that further surgery is invariably required to improve the cosmetic result, as the penis is often left lumpy rather than uniformly podgy.

Circumcision reversal

For men unhappy about having been circumcised as a child, there is now a non-surgical technique for restoring the foreskin, which relies on constant, gentle stretching of the skin on the shaft of the penis over the glans (head of the penis). Although this tissue-expansion technique might sound bizarre, it is commonly used in other forms of plastic or reconstructive surgery and is based on the methods practised by members of certain tribes to stretch their lips or earlobes.

The main complaint from men who have been circumcised is that constant exposure of their glans results in its surface becoming tougher and a lot less sensitive. They also lose the additional sensation from contact between the glans and the foreskin as it slides back and forth during masturbation or intercourse.

While it is possible to replace the foreskin surgically using a skin graft, this stretching of the penile skin is attractive to some men because it is seen as being more natural and, done properly, it should not be painful. However, the procedure requires considerable dedication, taking as long as three years before the glans becomes fully covered, depending on the tightness of the original circumcision. Information is available from NORM UK★ and also from the Uncircumcising Information Resources Centre★ in California.

Chapter 5

Fatherhood – a survival guide

IT DOESN'T matter whether you have been planning to become a father for months or years, or if the news that your partner is expecting has come as a complete shock, your reaction is bound to include a mixture of emotions, such as pride, excitement and anxiety. Having a baby with someone can dramatically change your life. It will certainly require some adjustments to your relationship, as there is now going to be another person around who needs love and attention from both of you. Yet, for many couples, the experience of parenthood adds more meaning and depth to their lives, despite all the additional worries and responsibilities.

Inevitably, some men worry whether they are really ready to be fathers. It is not only the financial implications of bringing up children – perhaps with the loss of one of the parents' income and all those extra expenses – that is worrying. Society now expects the father to do a lot more than just enjoy the fun that led to the conception and boast at work and in the pub about his children's achievements. This chapter is intended to help you through the minefield of modern fatherhood.

Health tips before conception

For couples planning to start a family, it is a good idea for both prospective parents to change to a more healthy lifestyle to reduce the risk of birth defects. A number of useful measures can also be taken by a man to improve the health of his sperm and thus increase the chance of his partner conceiving (see also infertility, pages 144–6). Remember that each sperm takes about ten weeks to develop and that it can be damaged at any time over this period.

Health tips

Stop smoking   A man who smokes tends to produce fewer sperm and have larger numbers of damaged sperm, which can impair his fertility. If a woman smokes while she is pregnant, she is more likely to go into premature labour, more likely to have complications during childbirth, and her baby's growth can be restricted. By giving up smoking together, couples have a much greater chance of the woman becoming pregnant and having a healthy child.

If either parent is still smoking, or starts again once the baby is born, there is an increased risk that the child will suffer from recurrent chest infections or asthma.

Cut down on alcohol   Regular heavy drinking may reduce the number of sperm a man produces, as well as damaging them, thereby lowering the chance of conception. Also, if a woman drinks heavily while she is pregnant, particularly in the first few weeks, she is more likely to miscarry or have a baby born with various abnormalities, including mental retardation. Cutting down on alcohol together will make it easier for your partner to succeed.

Eat a healthy diet   A lack of vitamins and minerals can interfere with sperm production and with the growth of a baby in the womb. Healthy eating habits are important throughout life, but particularly for your partner from the moment she becomes pregnant.

Exercise regularly   Your partner will find pregnancy and childbirth easier to cope with if she is physically fit to start with. If you exercise together, your health will benefit as well.

Practice relaxation   Couples who are stressed, particularly if the source of their worries is a failure to conceive as quickly as expected, often succeed in starting a family once they stop trying so hard and allow their love-making to be spontaneous and relaxed.

Keep your testicles cool   Anything that raises the temperature of your testicles can reduce sperm production: for example, being overweight or wearing tight underpants or trousers. Wear cotton boxer shorts and, if you have a paunch, take steps to lose weight (see pages 70–3).

Sperm problems Exposure to radiation and certain chemicals can impair fertility by damaging sperm. If these risks apply to your work, always follow safety guidelines.

If there is any inherited condition in your or your partner's family, such as sickle cell anaemia or Huntington's chorea, it is a good idea to receive genetic counselling before you start a family to establish the odds of your children being affected. Also, if any of your or your partner's relatives have been ill as young adults, or developed a serious illness before the age of 50, you should try to find out whether an inherited disorder might have been responsible.

Men who are HIV-positive are usually discouraged from having children, because of the risk of the baby, as well as their partner, becoming infected with the virus. However, a new technique has been developed in Italy, whereby the ejaculated sample is washed to remove the semen (which will be contaminated with HIV) and then any remaining HIV-infected cells are separated from the sperm. The sample of sperm is then artificially inseminated into the female partner. This technique, which reduces but does not completely eliminate the risk of passing on the HIV infection, is now available in a few hospitals in the UK.

Your partner's pregnancy

Being pregnant can cause a variety of minor complaints, such as back pain, indigestion, constipation and difficulty sleeping. Most women become irritable and very tired at times, particularly in the early and late stages of pregnancy, and your partner may want more attention paid to her and her needs than she did before she became pregnant.

To help you become more understanding and better prepared to make the necessary adjustments to your life while your partner is pregnant, it is a good idea to find out what pregnancy really involves in terms of the physical and emotional changes. Even if you are one of the few men who are unwilling or unable to attend the occasional antenatal class, you can still learn a great deal about pregnancy from the various good books that have been written on the subject.

Go with your partner when she has to attend the antenatal clinic, not necessarily to every appointment, but particularly at any time when there are specific worries or problems. That way you will be confirming to your partner that you are taking part in the pregnancy, showing interest and offering invaluable support. If there was a problem with the birth of a previous child, go together to talk to the staff who attended, or who are aware of the circumstances, so you can be reassured about what really happened and whether there are likely to be difficulties next time around.

Encourage your partner to discuss openly any anxieties she might have about the pregnancy and impending delivery. The more support you can give, the stronger your relationship will become. However, don't neglect to express your own fears and needs. You may even suffer a few pregnancy symptoms yourself, in sympathy, although any nausea, indigestion and difficulty sleeping are likely to be stress-related.

There are three main stages of pregnancy, known as trimesters, each stage three months long and characterised by specific changes in the mother and her baby:

First trimester

The embryo grows to about 5cm long and all its major organs develop. The mother will typically notice her breasts beginning to swell and they will often feel tender.

During this early stage of pregnancy, you must be prepared for your partner to complain of extreme tiredness at times and for her mood to vary suddenly from one day to the next. If your partner is suffering from morning sickness, you can help relieve this symptom by bringing her dry toast or biscuits, mineral water or weak tea first thing each morning.

You may also have to adjust your eating habits and, if you don't already do so, take a more active part in the cooking, as strong odours may aggravate your partner's nausea at all times, not just in the mornings.

Second trimester

This is often described as the blooming stage of pregnancy, because most women feel fit, healthy and full of energy at this time. Your partner may start to resent your attempts to offer help and support about the house, protesting about your apparent desire to treat her like an invalid, so be prepared to back off a little.

Women usually put on over half of their total pregnancy weight gain over these three months, with the baby growing rapidly and the uterus swelling upwards to cause the abdomen to distend. Your partner may have an increased appetite at this time, but she should not be eating for two. The actual increase in demand for food energy is only around 300 calories a day, so encourage your partner to fill herself up on high-nutrient, low-calorie snacks (see page 65).

Third trimester

During the final three months, many women again begin to feel tired as the delivery draws closer; now you should make even more effort to help out with everyday chores like shopping and ironing. Your partner may also start to worry about giving birth, so be prepared to talk through these worries.

A variety of complaints can develop, including breathlessness, swollen ankles, back pain, feeling faint and frequent need to pass urine. Getting comfortable in bed will also become more difficult, so find some extra pillows and cushions to support your partner in a more upright position.

Sex during pregnancy

Many women find that their sex drive is reduced during pregnancy. There are a number of possible reasons for this. First, your partner may be anxious about the changes in her body shape and feel that she is no longer attractive to you. It is therefore important to be tactful and reassuring, and to continue to demonstrate your physical attraction to her through kissing and cuddling, even when this is not going to lead to full intercourse.

Another barrier to sex may be the fear that penetration may injure the baby, introduce an infection, or lead to premature labour. Some women believe the myth that if they have an orgasm, this will in some way damage the baby.

There is certainly no evidence that sexual intercourse or orgasm can harm the baby and, as long as the man is not carrying any sexually transmitted disease, there should be no risk of infection to the mother or child. It has been suggested that sexual intercourse in late pregnancy, with the man on top, may occasionally hasten the onset of labour, sometimes by causing premature rupture of the membranes. However, this does not appear to happen with other sexual positions, which are usually more comfortable for her anyway.

Sex can normally continue throughout pregnancy, but remember your partner's breasts are likely to be tender during the first few weeks and, for the sake of comfort, you may have to use a side-to-side or rear-entry position in the third trimester. Circumstances in which sexual intercourse will have to cease include the onset of abdominal pain or vaginal bleeding at any stage of pregnancy, when medical advice should be sought. The doctor may advise a woman not to have sexual intercourse if she has a history of previous miscarriages, or there is a continuing threat of premature labour.

Attending the birth

No man should feel obliged to attend the birth of his baby, although those fathers who have witnessed the event usually describe it as a rewarding experience and say they feel much closer to their baby as a result.

Often the man has a false perception about how much blood and suffering is actually involved and, once he has been reassured, he is likely to be far happier about being there. Of course, your partner may not actually want you there, in which case you should respect her wishes.

Having agreed to attend the birth, you should find out more about labour – either from books or by attending the antenatal classes – so you can provide useful support. Discuss the birth plan with your partner, so you are aware of her wishes regarding issues such as pain relief and holding the baby immediately it is born.

Make sure your partner knows how to contact you at all times from at least the 36th week of pregnancy onwards, and if you plan to drive her to the hospital have a trial run to check the route and timing.

In addition to providing emotional support and helping pass time in the early stages, you can assist your partner in labour in many other ways:

- you can act as a guide and interpreter – many women find it difficult to keep track of what is happening around them and don't take in everything that is being said
- you can provide extra nursing care, giving your partner regular sips of water, mopping her brow with a damp flannel, gently rubbing her abdomen during a contraction, massaging her back to ease discomfort and helping her change position
- you can remind her about her breathing and relaxation exercises, to relieve the tension of each contraction, and encourage her when the time comes to push.

The new baby

You should be prepared for your partner and new baby to come home within the first three days after the delivery, sometimes sooner. Over these first few days, a new mother will need a great deal of support. She is likely to feel uncomfortable, with bruising and possibly stitches from the birth and her nipples may be sore if she is breastfeeding. Even if the baby is being bottle-fed, the mother's breasts are bound to become tender and engorged with milk.

Your partner needs to be given as much opportunity as possible to rest and catch up with her sleep. Childbirth is an exhausting process and the new baby will initially be demanding a feed every few hours, day and night.

Certainly, it is a good idea to be at home with your new baby for the first week or so, not just to offer support, but also to allow you to get more involved and thus avoid feeling left out. Don't be surprised if you feel frightened about taking responsibility for your baby, even if it is only for an hour while your partner takes a nap. Although some antenatal classes do include lessons in how to hold a baby and how to do things like change nappies, bathe, dress and feed your baby before he or she actually arrives on the scene, a lot of these tasks will simply have to be learnt as you go along. If you watch your partner, you will soon pick up the basics and, in every minute you spend alone with your baby, you will learn more about his or her needs and become more confident.

Unfortunately, many fathers do not make the effort to get involved and, as a result, start to feel lonely, jealous and rejected. Rather than openly discussing his anxiety and anger, the father finds an escape by burying himself in work or spending more time out with friends. His partner, in turn, then becomes annoyed about his attitude and lack of support. To avoid this breakdown in communication, ask your partner what help she needs and make it known that you want to be shown how to do all the different tasks relating to the care of the baby.

One particularly important job for the father is to help out with the other children if this baby is not the first. There are bound to be some feelings of jealousy towards this intruder, which are understandable but need to be defused. Encourage your older children to get involved with the new baby, but don't force them. While the new baby is being showered with attention and gifts from all your family and friends, take time out to show your love and affection for the others and give them a treat or present; the mother should also spend time alone with her older children, leaving Dad to take care of the new baby.

Coping with a crying baby

All babies cry when they need something: it is the only way they can call out for help. Over the first two weeks of life, the average baby cries for up to two hours a day, which reduces to one hour a day after the age of three months. Your baby may cry more than this, even though he or she is perfectly healthy.

Every baby has a unique range of cries which you and your partner will soon learn to recognise, including a hunger cry, a wet nappy cry, a tired cry, a temper cry and a pain cry. You should start by going to your baby promptly each time, to show that you are there when you are needed. Always handle the baby smoothly so he or she feels at ease in your arms.

Hunger is the usual reason for crying; a new baby may want milk every two hours at first. If a baby cries soon after a feed, this may be due to colic, in which case the baby will typically pull its legs up, scream and go red in the face. For colic, try rubbing your baby's tummy and gently bend and straighten its legs. A teaspoonful of gripe water or a colic remedy from the pharmacist containing activated dimethicone may also help.

Some babies need a lot of attention and cry because they are bored. Therefore, make sure your baby has a mobile or pictures to look at, or a toy to hold. A baby chair lets the baby watch what is going on, but don't put this chair anywhere unsafe or unsteady.

Alternatively, your baby might not like too much attention and may be easily startled. The best way to calm him or her is with cuddling and gentle rocking, talking or singing quietly, or playing music.

If your baby won't settle down to sleep, you can attempt to solve this problem in a number of ways:

- if you are working, don't come home and immediately start a lively game which gets your child over-excited. There should be a bedtime routine which calms your child down for the night. Even very young children enjoy a bedtime story
- if baby wakes in the night, give a feed, change the nappy if necessary, but don't have the main light on and do not play or make a lot of noise

- some babies settle more quickly if they are given a dummy to suck on, but don't dip this in milk or fruit juice or give your baby a drink as a comforter as the sugar will rot the teeth, even before they have broken through
- make sure the baby's room is not too hot or cold and that the curtains shut out the light properly. You can warm the pram or cot with a hot water bottle, but take it out before putting the baby down
- having positioned your baby on his or her back, wrap the covers firmly around to make him or her feel secure, but avoid overheating by not putting too much bedding on, and leave one arm free if your baby likes to suck his or her hand or fingers. Also position your baby with his or her feet down against the bottom of the cot to reduce the risk of the covers going over his or her head
- be prepared to allow your baby to cry for a few minutes; it is quite common for babies to cry as they are settling down to fall asleep
- if your child keeps calling out, go through the settling-down process again, but try not to take the baby out of the cot or pram unless you really have to
- the noise of a vacuum cleaner appears to get some babies off to sleep, but make sure it doesn't overheat if you have to leave it on
- a ride in the pram or car is another way to settle your baby, but it is not a good idea to make this a habit
- don't hesitate to take your baby into bed with you if that is the only way you are all going to get some sleep, unless of course you are under the influence of drink or drugs, in which case might you roll on top of him or her.

Controlling your temper

Parents whose baby won't stop crying may soon find that the love they have for their child turns to anger and frustration. The constant crying exhausts their patience and leaves them nervy and irritable.

First, it is important to realise that you can safely leave your baby crying. It won't cause any harm unless the baby has some medical problem, like a heart condition or a hernia. So put the baby out of earshot in another part of the house for a few minutes to give yourself the chance to unwind. If you are able to relax, this will help calm your baby when you return.

If you are afraid of losing control, find someone else you can trust to do the comforting and take your baby out. Don't be left alone with your baby if you can't cope with the crying. Call CRY-SIS★ if you need advice and support.

Any baby who seems to be crying excessively should be checked out by the health visitor or doctor. There may be a treatable cause, such as an allergy or infection.

Understanding the 'baby blues'

Giving birth and caring for a new baby are events that are emotionally as well as physically stressful. It is therefore hardly surprising that most women start to feel tired and tearful a few days after the delivery. Don't be surprised if your partner suddenly cries for no apparent reason, complains of feeling unable to cope, or says she is afraid she won't be able to take proper care of the baby. This is a common reaction to childbirth, which is popularly referred to as the 'baby blues'.

It is only when these feelings last longer than a couple of weeks, become severe enough to disrupt relationships in the home or begin to threaten the baby's welfare that a diagnosis of postnatal depression is made and treatment from a doctor is required.

To help your partner through the baby blues and reduce the risk of her becoming more severely depressed:

- get the house prepared before the baby's arrival
- make sure she has enough support over the first few weeks
- don't allow too many visitors at once
- ask for extra help from family and friends if you need it, for example, to babysit while you go out together
- encourage your partner to talk about her feelings
- suggest she joins a local parent and baby group.

The risk of postnatal depression is greater if there is some other source of stress, such as money worries or illness affecting the baby. Also, women who have suffered from depression before, even if it was unrelated to childbirth, are more likely to develop serious postnatal depression. However, there are some women who become depressed for months after having a baby, for which the only explanation is the hormonal changes that occur around this time.

If your partner is suffering from postnatal depression, the doctor will usually prescribe antidepressants and may also refer her for psychotherapy. Only a few extremely severe cases require admission to hospital to stop the mother harming herself or her baby.

Sex after childbirth

For at least the first two weeks, it will rarely be possible to resume normal sexual relations. Your partner will be far too sore owing to the bruising, scratches or small tears in the lining of her vagina and vulva, and she may have had stitches too. Also, sex would be messy because of the blood-stained discharge (lochia) that continues to drain from the uterus for some time after childbirth.

However, even if it is too soon to start having sex again, it is important to continue showing physical love and affection towards your partner with kisses and cuddles. Sex does not always have to include penetration or genital stimulation – there are other ways to make each other feel wanted and other erogenous zones on the body.

As the vagina and vulva heal, the soreness should soon ease off and the lochia will normally have cleared within a couple of weeks. Your partner may than decide she is ready to try sexual intercourse, but remember to take things slowly and gently at first.

About four in every ten women still feel uncomfortable six weeks after the delivery. This may be due to persistent bruising and inflammation, or there may be stitching that is a little tight. Also, some women notice they are dryer than they used to be, due to a reduction in vaginal secretions, particularly if they are breastfeeding, as a result of the change in hormone levels this causes. Your doctor may recommend a lubricant, but check to see if it is water-based, as oil-based lubricants may weaken a condom if that is the method of contraception you are using. Usually, all the discomfort during sex will have disappeared within three months; only a few women require some form of corrective surgery.

Because of the stretching of the tissues that occurs during a vaginal delivery, there will inevitably be loss of muscle tone in the vagina and some loss of sensation during intercourse as a result, for both you and your partner. This may be more of a problem if stitches have been put in too loosely. Sensation should return to normal over the first few months, as the vaginal muscles regain their tone, helped by your partner remembering to do her pelvic floor muscle exercises regularly each day. Again, a few women may require corrective surgery.

Research into sexual behaviour has shown that one in three mothers are having sex again within six weeks of the birth and the majority have resumed sexual intercourse by three months. However, over half of these women reported that they initially had less interest in sex than before.

There are a number of reasons why women are less keen on sex after childbirth. First, it is important to appreciate just how tiring looking after a baby can be. At the end of the day, most new mothers just about have the energy to collapse into bed. Another common concern is the fear of falling pregnant again, so make sure you have agreed on a reliable method of contraception. Pregnancy can happen even before your partner has had her first normal period after the birth – don't believe the myth that she can't get pregnant while she is still breastfeeding.

Within a year most women start enjoying sex again as much as they did before the pregnancy. The key to preserving your love and affection for each other, despite any initial sexual difficulties, is to try to talk openly and honestly about these problems. You can't expect good sex if the rest of your relationship is not going smoothly. It takes a while to adjust to having a new member of the family and, if you are to stop a gap opening up between you and your partner, you need to make the time and the effort to discuss and resolve each new difficulty as it arises.

Be sensitive towards your partner's feelings about her own physical attractiveness, but also encourage her to do all her postnatal exercises every day, especially those designed to strengthen her pelvic floor muscles. Don't expect her figure to return to normal at once: it may take many weeks for the muscles in her abdomen to become firm again. As a result of the breast changes that occur normally during pregnancy, her breasts may end up smaller and less firm than before.

The father's role

Children need to be able to relate to their father. Although he may be working hard to provide the necessary financial support for his partner and children, he must also spend 'quality time' at home to build a relationship with his family.

Children tend to see their father as a role model. They may not appear to take much notice of what he says to them, but they are strongly influenced by his behaviour and attitudes. How the father handles a particular problem sets an example to the child, affecting the way the child responds in a similar situation.

Children are constantly seeking to gain their father's approval and respect, which is why it is important to become involved in their achievements at school and at play. Unfortunately, there is a risk that parents will start to use a child's performance to satisfy their own previously unfulfilled ambitions, which may lead to their pushing the child too hard, or for the wrong reasons. If this starts to happen, both parents need to step back and remember that children deserve unconditional love and support, regardless of success or failure.

Parents of a child who has been having problems at school, for example bullying, may not realise, through no fault of their own, that anything is wrong. There is no easy answer to this. You simply need to keep an eye and ear out for clues and create an atmosphere in your home in which your children feel they can approach you with their difficulties without worrying that they are letting you down by not being able to sort things out for themselves. However, it is not a good idea to pester children with questions. Simply give them the time and opportunity to speak out and then listen to what they have to say.

It is important that you and your partner are consistent in the way you discipline your children. If you do smack a child, it should not be for something trivial, not be hard enough to cause injury and not just be an outlet for your lack of patience or frustration. Any time you feel the urge to lash out, walk away to give yourself time to calm down.

Living with a teenager

Few teenagers pass through their adolescence without at least some emotional or psychological upset, as they struggle to find their own social identity and come to terms with new desires that they may initially be unable to fulfil during the difficult transition into adulthood.

Adolescents will often challenge the authority figures and symbols in their lives, just as a normal part of trying to establish their independence. To help them identify with their friends and give them a sense of belonging, adolescents also tend to adopt the extreme styles of behaviour and dress of that particular group.

Here are a few guidelines to help you and your partner survive these turbulent years:

- try not to be upset by arguments. Remember they are a normal part of growing up and try to argue only over important issues
- listen to what your son or daughter has to say and try to reach a compromise. Although teenagers will generally ignore and even resent your advice, however sensible and tactfully worded, as they grow up they will become more receptive
- show an interest in their friends and leisure activities, but also respect their privacy
- be prepared to discuss sex openly
- ignore their appearance if you can – most teenagers eventually tone down their dress and behaviour on their own initiative
- agree on a reasonable curfew time, with a later hour allowed when there is no school or college the next day
- talk through feelings of anxiety or depression. Short episodes of depression in an adolescent are common, but prolonged depression needs medical help
- be on the lookout for signs of anorexia nervosa, such as always missing out on meals and an obsession with losing weight, which is often accompanied by excessive exercising; bulimia, in which bingeing is followed by vomiting, is also becoming more common
- be alert to the warning signs of drug or alcohol abuse, such as alternating periods of sleepiness and hyperactivity, sudden mood swings, shivering and slurred speech, articles and money disappearing from the house, but don't make this accusation unless you are convinced your suspicions are correct. Try to discuss the issues and risks (see pages 95–103) rather than laying down the law.

Chapter 6

A–Z of common health problems in men

THIS chapter explains not only disorders which are unique to men, but also a large number of conditions common to both sexes which are either medically serious or simply aggravating or embarrassing. This is not, of course, an encyclopaedia of every conceivable health problem.

The list is arranged in alphabetical order.

Acne

Acne is an extremely common skin complaint among adolescents. Mild cases are characterised by spots, whiteheads and blackheads appearing on the face, with a fresh crop of spots emerging as the older ones heal. In more severe cases, acne spreads to the skin on the chest, back and sometimes even the buttocks.

The cause of acne is an excessive build-up of sebum – the waxy substance produced by glands adjacent to the hair follicles which keeps the skin lubricated. As a result of this build-up, the channel that drains sebum to the skin surface may become blocked, causing the nearby follicle to swell and inflame, forming an angry-looking spot.

While the spot remains covered it is called a whitehead; if it opens up, exposure of the sebum to oxygen causes chemical changes, the spot darkens as a result and is popularly referred to as a blackhead. Occasionally, one or more of these spots may expand under pressure to form a cyst or abscess.

A number of factors can trigger or aggravate acne, the most important of which is the sudden increase in the production of male sex hormones around the time of puberty. These hormones, which women produce in small amounts as well, stimulate the release of sebum in addition to their influence on sexual development.

Accumulation of bacteria on the skin, high humidity, certain greasy cosmetics and a few prescription medicines can also play a part in this condition. However, acne is *not* caused by eating chocolate or fried food, masturbation or having dirty skin.

To minimise problems with acne:

- wash your face twice daily with a mild, unscented soap
- wash your hair frequently and keep it up off your forehead
- avoid any aftershave cream or lotion that might block the hair follicles
- do not pick or squeeze your spots
- ask your pharmacist to recommend an acne preparation: these can be very effective in mild cases.

See your doctor if:

- the above measures fail to help
- spots have appeared in places other than your face
- you have developed abscesses or cysts.

Your doctor may prescribe low doses of an antibiotic to reduce inflammation around the follicles and to kill off certain types of skin bacteria. A gel containing benzoyl peroxide is useful for unblocking the sebum channels, which it does by peeling off the outer layers of skin. Drainage of sebum can also be improved using a cream, gel or lotion derived from vitamin A, known as tretinoin.

This vitamin A drug is also available as isotretinoin capsules, which can be very effective at controlling severe acne and reducing the risk of the skin being left pitted or scarred. However, isotretinoin is a powerful drug that can only be prescribed under the supervision of a skin specialist and only with extreme caution because of the risk of liver damage.

Most sufferers grow out of acne in their early twenties and in those few cases where there is some residual scarring, a cosmetic medical procedure, such as gently shaving off the top layers of skin (dermabrasion), will usually help.

Agoraphobia

Agoraphobia is a fear of going into open, crowded or public places, such as shops or restaurants. Just the thought of leaving home or mixing with other people can cause feelings of severe anxiety or panic (see also 'Panic attacks'). Although this condition is less common in men than in women, it still interferes with the lives of many men in the UK.

In a mild form, agoraphobia may just prevent a man from using public transport or being in a crowd at a soccer game, for example. In extreme cases, however, the man may never leave the house.

This type of phobia often first comes on as a result of a stressful life-event, such as bereavement. The person may start to misuse alcohol or tranquillisers as a way of trying to relieve the associated anxiety symptoms. However, in some sufferers, alcohol or tranquilliser abuse might bring on the condition in the first place, as the withdrawal symptoms can cause the same sense of anxiety.

Treatment may include behavioural therapy, where the individual is helped to confront his fears in a controlled way while practising relaxation techniques, having psychotherapy, and/or taking an anti-depressant.

AIDS

See pages 125–8.

Alzheimer's disease

Alzheimer's disease is the most common cause of dementia in the UK. Although it may occasionally strike men in their forties or fifties, most sufferers are over 65 years old when symptoms, such as loss of short-term memory and disorientation, first begin. Dementia is not an inevitable feature of growing old. Many elderly men remain mentally and intellectually active throughout their lives.

In Alzheimer's disease, tiny areas of brain damage develop, consisting of plaques and tangles. Plaques form between brain cells and are made up of deposits of a protein called beta-amyloid. Tangles are abnormal, thread-like deposits of a protein called tau that form inside the brain cells. These changes make it harder for the brain cells to produce chemicals such as acetylcholine, which carry nerve messages to different parts of the brain.

The underlying cause of Alzheimer's disease remains unknown. Research to date has suggested that this condition may be related to a persistent viral infection in the brain, to poisoning from a build up of aluminium or to a genetic factor. Symptoms become progressively more severe until the man is too confused or withdrawn to be able to look after himself safely any more.

Any man developing symptoms or signs of dementia will undergo extensive tests to check that there is not some other treatable cause for his mental deterioration, such as anaemia, an underactive thyroid, a vitamin deficiency or depression.

Once the diagnosis of Alzheimer's disease is made, treatment will focus mainly on providing good nursing and social care, either to help the sufferer to be cared for at home or within a nursing home. However, a new class of drug – the anticholinesterases – which includes donepezil and rivastigmine, may also be prescribed, as they can help improve early symptoms relating to loss of memory and poor judgement in some mild to moderate cases, by reversing the decline in levels of the brain chemical acetylcholine.

In severe cases, where the sufferer has become aggressive or agitated, he may need to be given tranquillisers. Almost constant supervision may be required to prevent him coming to any harm. For further information and support, you can contact the Alzheimer's Disease Society.*

Angina

Angina (see also 'Heart attack', pages 233–5) is cramp of the heart muscle, causing a transient pain or tightness across the centre of the chest that sometimes spreads to the neck, jaw or arms. In some men, it may be a particular activity that brings on the pain, such as the exertion of climbing a flight of stairs, or eating a large meal. For others, angina may be provoked by stress, anger or extremes of temperature.

Descriptions of angina vary from a mild aching sensation to a heavy, crushing pain; sometimes the discomfort is mistaken for indigestion or heartburn. Other symptoms that often accompany an anginal attack include sweating, nausea, dizziness and difficulty in breathing.

Angina is caused by a lack of oxygen and nutrients reaching the heart muscle, usually because the coronary arteries which encircle and supply blood to the heart have become clogged up with fatty deposits – a condition known as atherosclerosis. This narrowing of the coronary arteries prevents the normal increase in blood flow that should occur when extra demands are placed on the heart, such as during exercise.

The risk of atherosclerosis increases with age, but there are a number of lifestyle factors which speed up the development of fatty deposits inside the arteries. These contributory factors include tobacco smoking, lack of exercise, excessive alcohol consumption and eating a lot of foods that contain large amounts of saturated fat and cholesterol.

Men may develop angina as early as their 30s or 40s, whereas women are protected from atherosclerosis by oestrogen until the menopause, when there is a sudden decline in the production of this female sex hormone.

To confirm a diagnosis of angina, the doctor will normally carry out an electrocardiogram (ECG), which is a recording of the electrical activity passing through the heart muscle.

Treatment of angina includes using drugs to widen the coronary arteries (nitrates, calcium channel blockers, potassium channel activators) and drugs which reduce the heart's demand for oxygen by slowing the heart rate (betablockers). Surgical procedures such as angioplasty (insertion of a catheter with an inflatable balloon tip into the narrowed arteries to flatten the fatty deposits) or bypass grafting (attachment of a blood vessel to redirect blood flow around the blockage) successfully relieve angina symptoms in many people.

Self-help measures for angina sufferers include:

- stopping smoking
- exercising regularly, but only until the symptoms come on
- relaxation measures to reduce stress
- avoiding exercise on hot or very cold days, or soon after a meal
- losing excess weight to put less strain on the heart.

Anorexia nervosa

Although anorexia nervosa, popularly referred to as 'slimmer's disease', affects mainly teenage girls and young women, it is important to be aware that some young men are also vulnerable to this compulsive eating disorder, particularly men working as models or ballet dancers.

This condition is characterised by a fear of putting on weight; the victim typically has a distorted body image and sees himself as being fatter than he really is. As a result, he deliberately starves himself and may also exercise obsessively.

In addition to being abnormally thin, the sufferer may become weak and tired and, due to hormonal changes, develop fine downy hair over his whole body. Left untreated, he could die from the effects of starvation, for example from a cardiac arrest due to a lack of potassium.

Treatment often requires admission to hospital to take part in a supervised re-feeding programme as, left alone, the anorectic is likely to hide or throw away food to avoid eating. To reduce the risk of a relapse, long-term psychotherapy, family counselling and sometimes an anti-depressant, may be given. However, as many as 50 per cent of men treated for anorexia nervosa go on having symptoms for many years.

Anxiety

The main causes of anxiety in men, both young and old, are worries about health, money and unemployment. People who have been involved in some sort of serious accident or incident (being attacked, for example) may develop a form of anxiety known as post-traumatic stress disorder in which they continue to feel anxious long after the event and its implications are over.

While anxiety is a perfectly normal reaction to any problem or fear that cannot readily be resolved, it may become a disorder in its own right if it is so intense or prolonged that it prevents the individual from thinking clearly or rationally, sleeping properly, or coping with everyday activities.

Psychological symptoms related to anxiety may include difficulty concentrating, irritability, being easily distracted, getting tired easily but having trouble falling asleep at night, loss of appetite and a sense of impending doom. Some of the more common physical symptoms are palpitations, muscle tension, trembling, sweating and a feeling of suffocation. Mistaking these symptoms for a physical illness only serves to make the anxiety worse.

Self-help measures to relieve anxiety include:

- talking about the problem to a trusted friend, neighbour or relative who is a good listener and whose opinions you respect; sharing worries and feelings can put them into a calmer perspective
- talking to someone who has been through a similar experience, for example, by contacting the appropriate self-help group
- relaxation exercises, regular physical activities and meditation (see Chapter 3); if you know you tend to be anxious, try practising a relaxation technique regularly, not just when a crisis is already underway.

If symptoms of anxiety persist or recur despite these measures, it is important to seek professional help. According to the Royal College of Psychiatrists, prolonged or severe anxiety is only rarely due to any significant mental illness, so there is no need to be scared of seeing a doctor. It is certainly better to receive treatment early, rather than late, and you are extremely unlikely to be carted off to hospital against your will.

Your GP may decide to refer you for psychotherapy (see Glossary) to help you identify, understand and come to terms with the underlying reasons for the anxiety, which are often not immediately apparent. Treatment may last for several weeks or even months.

Tranquillisers can also be very effective as a short-term measure, but do not deal with the root cause of the anxiety and are not helpful in the long term because of the risk of addiction. Nowadays, doctors are advised to prescribe tranquillisers only for a brief period to help someone through an acute crisis. If they are taken regularly for longer than a couple of weeks there is a risk of addiction, with unpleasant withdrawal symptoms when the drug is stopped or the dose is reduced too quickly.

Appendicitis

The most common surgical emergency in the UK, appendicitis (inflammation of the appendix) affects about one in every 500 people each year. Although it may strike men at any age, it is most likely to occur between the ages of 15 and 24 years old.

Why the appendix, the worm-like tube that branches off the large bowel, should become inflamed is usually unknown. However, one cause may be that a small pellet of faeces has obstructed it.

Typically, appendicitis begins as a vague discomfort in the centre of the abdomen which, after a few hours, becomes a much more severe, sharp pain that localises on the lower right-hand side. Additional symptoms may include slight fever, loss of appetite, nausea and vomiting.

Anyone who suffers from persistent abdominal pain lasting longer than a few hours should seek immediate medical attention, either from his GP or the hospital accident and emergency department. Diagnosis from physical examination can be difficult because there are many other possible causes of right-sided abdominal pain, such as enlarged lymph glands from a viral infection, inflammation of the bowel or a kidney infection.

Because of the risk of the inflamed appendix perforating to cause peritonitis, which, in turn, can cause serious complications, if the doctor has any doubt, the individual is likely to be admitted for surgery.

Asthma

Asthma is a lung disease characterised by recurrent attacks of breathlessness that are usually accompanied by wheezing, tightness in the chest and a cough. The individual finds it difficult to breathe in and even more difficult to breathe out. Attacks often occur at night or in the early hours of the morning. Children with asthma may not show any signs of wheezing but will usually cough, especially at night and also when they laugh or run around.

The symptoms of asthma are caused by narrowing of the bronchi (airways) in the lungs, due to a tightening of the muscles in the walls of the bronchi (see page 18). There is also an increased production of mucus in the bronchi, which further interferes with the normal flow of air in and out of the lungs.

Asthma attacks can start at any age and may be brought on by a variety of different factors, including colds and 'flu, sudden strenuous exercise, breathing in cold air, an allergic reaction to pollen, mould, dust, feathers or fur, and stress or anxiety. For some people, however, there are no obvious causes that can be avoided.

To confirm the diagnosis, the doctor will usually arrange lung-function tests: for example, asking the individual to breathe out forcefully into a machine which measures the maximum air-flow speed. Sometimes this machine has to be taken home so that readings can be repeated at those times when the symptoms come on or worsen. Asthmatics have an abnormally low peak flow, particularly in the evening, in the early hours of the morning and during an attack.

Treatment of asthma consists firstly of a bronchodilator, which relieves symptoms by widening the airways. Many asthma patients also receive additional medication (usually a corticosteroid) which, by reducing the underlying inflammation, helps keep the disease under control, lowering the frequency and severity of attacks. Both the 'reliever' and the 'preventer' drugs are usually inhaled from a pressurised aerosol or a similar device.

A new type of drug, known as an antileukotriene, has recently become available as an add-on therapy to the bronchodilator and corticosteroid inhalers, for those asthmatics still troubled by symptoms. This drug, which is taken by mouth, reduces the inflammation caused by leukotrienes inside the airways.

Self-help measures for asthma sufferers include:

- never smoking; staying out of smoky atmospheres
- reducing exposure to dust mites by having someone else do regular vacuum-cleaning, dusting with a damp cloth, washing the curtains every few weeks, vacuum-cleaning the mattress and covering it with plastic, and using a mite-killing spray
- taking regular exercise, using the 'reliever' inhaler before starting
- asking your doctor for appropriate 'preventive' medication if your symptoms are interfering with your life by stopping normal activities or waking you at night
- having a 'flu jab every autumn.

See your doctor as soon as possible if your 'reliever' medication stops being effective, or if you are having to use it more often. You should call for emergency help if you or the person you are caring for becomes severely breathless (for example, to the extent that it makes talking difficult), or if the skin becomes pale, clammy or turns blue. Most deaths from asthma are associated with a delay in calling the doctor.

Athlete's foot

Athlete's foot is an unsightly and irritating fungal infection that affects the skin of the feet. It usually starts between and underneath the toes, but can sometimes spread to the undersurface of the feet. Symptoms include itching and soreness of the skin, which may burn and then start to crack and peel. In some cases, the infected skin turns white, becomes inflamed and weepy, or begins to smell unpleasant.

The fungi which cause it – usually dermatophytes – feed off the protein-rich material (keratin) from the top layers of skin. Fungi are transferred from one person to another within the fragments of dead skin that are continually being shed from the feet.

Because the athlete's foot fungi prefer to grow in warm, moist surroundings, this condition is more likely to occur in people who don't dry properly between their toes. Two ways in which the infection may easily be picked up are when someone dries himself on a damp towel already used by someone who has athlete's foot, or by walking barefoot across a damp, contaminated floor, for example in a communal shower, changing room or swimming pool.

Any man who uses communal bathing facilities regularly, such as swimmers and others who play sports, stands an increased chance of acquiring this infection, but it doesn't affect athletes alone: the fungi can be just as easily transferred in the family bathroom.

About 10 per cent of the population are thought to be suffering from athlete's foot at any one time, although, for some unknown reason, some people seem to be resistant to this condition. Athlete's foot is more common in adults than in children and is usually picked up for the first time during the teen years. Men are more likely to develop athlete's foot, partly because of the closed, heavier shoes they wear, which encourage sweaty feet.

Self-help measures to combat athlete's foot include:

- drying the feet carefully, paying particular attention to the skin between the toes; using a separate foot towel helps prevent the fungi spreading to other parts of the body, such as the groin,
- using your own towel and bath mat to protect other people who share your bathroom
- wearing socks made of natural materials (like cotton), rather than synthetics (such as nylon), which don't absorb sweat efficiently
- changing socks daily, and more often if you have sweaty feet
- wearing shoes with ventilation holes or a porous upper. Open-toe sandals are ideal but not practical for outdoor wear in wet or cold weather
- avoiding shoes which are a tight fit and which cramp your toes together
- not wearing the same pair of shoes on consecutive days: it can take at least 24 hours for them to air and dry out properly
- asking your pharmacist for an antifungal preparation and using it as instructed, which may be twice a day for four weeks or for at least ten days after the skin has cleared
- washing your hands after applying treatment to prevent the infection spreading to other areas of the body
- wearing protective shoes such as flip-flops in showers, changing rooms and around swimming pools.

See your doctor if the infection doesn't clear up or keeps coming back. You may need a more powerful antifungal drug that is available only on prescription. You should also seek medical help if the infection spreads to the nails, causing them to crumble or become discoloured.

Back pain

Back pain is the most common reason why people take sick leave from work. It is often accompanied by sciatica – pain radiating down the back of the thigh and leg – due to irritation of one or more of the spinal nerves. The different causes of and treatments for sciatica are the same as those for back pain.

In the majority of cases, back pain is brought on by excessive strain on the lower spine, resulting, for example, from poor posture, being overweight, or doing a lot of heavy lifting and carrying. This strain may cause damage in the form of torn ligament or muscle fibres, displacement of some of the joints between adjacent vertebrae, or even a prolapsed disc, where part of the spongy material between two vertebrae is protruding and pressing on a nearby ligament or nerve.

Often an acute (sudden) episode of back pain clears up with bed rest and painrelievers before any investigations are carried out, so the exact cause may never be identified. However, if back pain is particularly severe or persists after 48 hours of taking painrelievers and lying flat, you should see a doctor. Immediate medical attention is essential if there are also symptoms of pressure on a spinal nerve, such as weakness, pins and needles, numbness or loss of bladder or bowel control.

Your doctor may prescribe strong painrelievers and muscle relaxants. Imaging of the spine may be done with X-rays, magnetic resonance imaging (an imaging technique using a powerful magnetic field and pulses of radiowaves) or CT scanning, where a detailed cross-section of the spine is produced using multi-angled X-ray beams under computerised control.

If there is only minor damage to the back, your doctor may recommend traction or manipulation, both of which can be extremely effective in relieving pain and muscle spasm in some cases. More serious conditions such as a stress fracture or a spondylolithesis (vertebra slipping forwards) may require surgery.

Other possible causes of back pain include osteoarthritis, ankylosing spondylitis (inflammation of vertebral joints), osteoporosis and, rarely, cancer.

Self-help measures to prevent or reduce back pain include:

- using a firm mattress, or placing a board under your mattress, to provide support at night
- losing excess weight to reduce load on the spine
- doing exercises to strengthen spinal and abdominal muscles, such as swimming
- using a heating pad or portable massager to relax muscle spasm
- wearing a lumbar support (helps some people)
- adopting the correct posture when sitting or lifting.

Sitting properly The chair should be adjusted to a height where your feet can be flat on the ground and knees level with or slightly above your hips. The seat should support three-quarters of the back of your thighs without digging in behind your knees. The work surface should be at elbow height.

Lifting safely Stand close to the object. Bend your knees, keep your back straight (but not uncomfortably so) and slowly rise, taking the load through your leg muscles.

Bad breath

Many people worry about having bad breath, but only a few actually suffer from this embarrassing problem. If you think your breath smells unpleasant, then pluck up the courage to ask someone close to you to sniff out the truth. Unfortunately, it is difficult to test your own breath, although occasionally you can tell by licking and then sniffing the back of your hand.

It is not uncommon to wake in the morning with a dry mouth accompanied by a stale odour. This is due to a reduction in the amount of saliva you produce while you are asleep, and tends to be worse if you breathe through your mouth, smoke, or drank a lot of alcohol the night before. A soft coating forms over the tongue and teeth and this begins to be broken down by healthy bacteria in the mouth to release chemicals which smell foul. As soon as you clean your teeth, the coating and the odour should disappear.

If you follow a few simple measures, you should be able to keep your breath fresh during the day. Eat regular meals, as chewing and swallowing boost your production of saliva, which acts as a natural mouthwash to clean and freshen your breath. Between meals, you can use sugar-free chewing gum or mints, a piece of fresh fruit or a raw vegetable to stimulate the flow of saliva. Also, make sure you drink enough fluids to keep your mouth moist.

Certain foods can produce a distinctive odour on your breath, which won't go away for several hours, whatever you do to try to mask the smell. Foods such as garlic and onions, once they have been digested, release sulphur-containing chemicals which get carried in the bloodstream to the lungs; the sulphur then gets breathed out over anyone who gets close.

The most common cause of persistent bad breath is poor oral hygiene. It is important therefore to clean your teeth at least twice a day, preferably after meals. Use a toothbrush that is in good condition, and check with your dentist that you are using the correct brushing technique. Failure to remove particles of food from around your teeth, especially meat, fish and dairy products, will allow them time to start decomposing, with the release of foul-smelling chemicals. If you wear a denture, take it out before you go to bed; and keep it scrupulously clean by soaking it overnight, using a solution of sodium hypochlorite if it is made of acrylic, or chlorhexidine for metal.

Mouthwashes, freshener sprays and capsules are usually highly effective at masking bad breath. However, if you suffer from persistent bad breath, make an appointment to see your dentist; the usual reason is a rotten tooth or a gum infection that needs treatment. If your dentist is unable to find the cause, you should visit your doctor. Bad breath can sometimes be caused by a disease somewhere else in the body. Throat, sinus and lung infections, diabetes, kidney or liver disease, as well as certain medications, can all make your breath smell bad.

Body odour

Everyone has their own characteristic body odour. Most people have only a faint smell on their skin, which is often difficult to detect. Only when this smell becomes particularly strong or unpleasant should body odour be regarded as a problem. The fear of smelling offensive to others often drives many people to mask their natural smell, however mild it is.

Your body has roughly two million sweat glands and produces over three litres of sweat each day. Most of this sweat evaporates quickly. Hot weather, exercise and anxiety will all cause you to sweat more and when it is humid the sweat won't evaporate as efficiently, making you feel sticky and uncomfortable. Some people produce large amounts of sweat, however cool, relaxed and rested they are. Overweight people tend to sweat a lot because they are more likely to overheat.

Fresh sweat does not normally produce any unpleasant odour unless you have been eating garlic, onions, curry or other spicy foods. It is stale sweat that has been on your body or on your clothing for several hours that smells. This is because the bacteria that normally live on the surface of your skin release chemicals from the sweat that give off a pungent odour. Sweat tends to build up in areas where it cannot evaporate easily, such as under the arms and in the groin. These areas also produce a special type of sweat which is more likely to go stale because it contains fats and proteins which encourage bacteria to grow, whereas sweat from other parts of the body is mainly salt water with only small amounts of waste products in it. The reason why sweaty feet often smell so bad is that the bacteria that rot sweat thrive in warm, airless places, such as inside your socks.

Because body odour is usually due to the smell of stale sweat the best way to prevent it is to change your underpants and socks every day and to change your other clothes regularly. You should bathe or shower once a day and especially after exercise. But don't wash too obsessively as this can actually increase body odour by removing healthy skin bacteria. It is also important to dry properly as bacteria like living on moist skin. Some people find that applying talcum powder after a bath or shower helps keep their skin dry. If you tend to sweat a lot, wear comfortable, loose clothing and cotton rather than synthetics, so that your skin can breathe and the sweat can evaporate.

Using a scented talc to mask the smell of stale sweat may make the smell even worse. It is better to use a deodorant that contains an antiperspirant. Most antiperspirants work either by stopping bacteria from rotting the sweat, or by preventing the sweat from evaporating, which then holds the smell in. If you decide to try a new brand, only use a little at first in case you are sensitive to it.

If you are worried about body odour, see your doctor. If you have a sweat problem, he or she may recommend you wash with antiseptic or antibacterial soap and may prescribe an antiperspirant which contains aluminium chloride. This works by reducing the amount of sweat you produce, but because it can irritate the skin it is usually applied only to non-sensitive areas.

In very severe cases, an operation can be carried out to remove sweat glands from under the arms, but this often works for only a few months before the sweating returns.

Occasionally, body odour is caused by something other than stale sweat, such as fungal infection (e.g. athlete's foot) or an infected skin ulcer which needs special treatment. The smell may also be coming from somewhere other than the skin, for example, from bad breath due to tooth decay or gum disease, or from stale urine in an incontinent person.

Bronchitis

Bronchitis is a condition in which the main airways inside the lungs (bronchi) become inflamed (see page 18). As a result of this inflammation, the normal production of mucus (also referred to as sputum or phlegm) is increased and it often becomes discoloured. The typical symptom is a loose cough which brings up yellow or green sputum.

An acute (sudden) attack of bronchitis is usually due to either a viral or bacterial infection of the airways. In most people, it develops as a complication of a cold or 'flu, and other symptoms may include a fever, chest pains and breathlessness.

If you develop symptoms of acute bronchitis, see your doctor. You may be prescribed a course of antibiotics to deal with any bacterial infection present. Self-help measures include drinking plenty of fluids to help thin the mucus and taking an expectorant to make the sputum easier to cough up. But avoid cough suppressants such as codeine linctus as they will encourage a build up of mucus in the airways.

Using a steam vaporiser in your room, or inhaling steam, can help reduce congestion and make breathing feel easier, whereas spending time in a dry or smoky atmosphere will irritate the already sensitive airways, aggravating the cough as a result.

Sufferers from chronic (long-term) bronchitis have a productive cough on most days for three months or more every year. This is mainly a disease of smokers and those who have been exposed to high levels of air pollution. Apart from the persistent or recurrent cough, there may be wheezing, chest tightness and breathlessness on exertion.

Tobacco smoke and other air pollutants irritate the cells lining the bronchi, thereby increasing the production of thick, sticky mucus which clogs up these airways. When this irritation continues regularly over several years, there is a steady increase in the size and activity of the mucus-producing glands, which explains why the symptoms become prolonged and difficult to treat. Smoking also interferes with the normal process of clearing mucus, which is why smokers say they need a cigarette to help them cough to clear their lungs.

Stopping smoking and wearing a protective face mask in a polluted area can start to improve the condition at once. However, the longer the exposure has been going on, the more severe the damage is likely to be. Also, a chronic bronchitic becomes more susceptible to a bacterial infection, which will cause his symptoms to flare up – doctors call this acute-on-chronic bronchitis.

Self-help measures for chronic bronchitis are as described above for acute attacks. Antibiotics may be prescribed when a flare-up of symptoms is due to an infection. The doctor may also prescribe a bronchodilator, usually as an inhaler, to try to open up the obstructed airways, but this drug won't work as well for chronic bronchitis as it does for asthma.

If you are susceptible to attacks of acute bronchitis, or you suffer from chronic bronchitis, you should visit your doctor at the first signs of a cold or of 'flu going to your chest. People with chronic bronchitis are also advised to be routinely vaccinated against influenza each autumn, as a dose of 'flu could make their chest condition a lot more serious.

Bulimia

Bulimia is a compulsive eating disorder characterised by secretive episodes of uncontrolled over-eating, invariably followed by self-induced vomiting. As with anorexia nervosa, it is much less common in men than in women, but it still occurs in a significant number of young men and can have a damaging effect on both their physical and mental health.

In addition to the damage to teeth caused by repeated vomiting of stomach acids, bulimia can cause dehydration, weakness and cramps due to salt imbalance, kidney and liver damage. Also, bulimia is often accompanied by abuse of laxatives, which can interfere with normal bowel function.

Treatment includes a supervised eating programme, usually in hospital, along with psychotherapy or counselling. Because the sufferer can become extremely depressed by his compulsive behaviour, sometimes to the point of feeling suicidal, an anti-depressant may also be prescribed.

Bunions

A bunion is a firm pad of skin filled with fluid that has formed on the outside of the big toe, as a result of friction and pressure from a tight shoe. Bunions develop in people who have a deformity of the joint at the base of their big toe, causing this joint to protrude abnormally.

At first, the area of skin under pressure may thicken to form a callus or corn. Then, if the pressure persists, a fluid-filled sac will appear as the body's way of trying to cushion the skin and bone. It is this fluid-filled tissue that is referred to as a bunion.

The main cause of the big toe deformity is thought to be an inherited weakness in the ligaments that help support and shape the foot. However, wearing ill-fitting or badly designed shoes can also play a part. If the deformity is only slight, a corrective sock bought from the pharmacy may hold the toe straight. A chiropodist can remove any callus or corn that has formed, as well as provide you with a protective felt pad to reduce pressure over the bony prominence.

Once a bunion has formed, your doctor may inject the tender area with corticosteroid to ease the inflammation. However, if the deformity is unsightly or if the bunion remains tender and swollen, you may be referred for surgery to correct the deformity. Although surgery will leave you with a small scar along the back of the big toe, and a toe that is slightly shorter, plumper and more floppy than before, this is a small sacrifice to pay for getting rid of the pain and being able to look forward to your next visit to the shoe shop.

Cancer

Cancer is not just one disease. There are many different types, each of which involves unrestrained growth of cells inside a specific organ or tissue in the body. The most common types of cancer in men are lung, skin, large bowel, prostate and testicular cancer. Stomach, pancreas and bladder cancers are also important causes of death in men.

By being aware of the warning symptoms of cancer, regularly examining your skin and testicles for abnormal changes and visiting your doctor for an urgent check-up if you notice any of the warning signals, the diagnosis can be confirmed at the earliest possible stage, which will give subsequent treatment a greater chance of success. Do not be afraid of being made to look a fool by seeming to panic unnecessarily. Even though the symptoms will often be due to a harmless or non-cancerous condition which will readily respond to treatment, in those few cases where the diagnosis does turn out to be cancer, any delay in treatment reduces the likelihood of a successful outcome.

In recent years there have been a number of advances in cancer treatment, with improvements in surgical and radiotherapy techniques and a wider variety of powerful anticancer drugs. Men who delay seeking medical help could be missing out on potentially life-saving therapies.

Lung cancer

This is the commonest type of cancer in men by a long way, with over 80 new cases per 100,000 men diagnosed each year in the UK, and an annual death rate in men of over 25,000. The peak age for lung cancer is between 65 and 75 years; it is rare in men below the age of 40.

Cigarette smoking is the main cause of lung cancer. The more cigarettes smoked and the younger the age at which smoking started, the greater the risk. Cigar and pipe smokers have a lower chance of developing lung cancer, but their risk is still higher than for non-smokers.

Inhalation of tobacco smoke by non-smokers – known as passive smoking – has also been shown to be a risk factor for lung cancer. In addition, working with cancer-causing substances like asbestos may cause certain types of lung cancer, especially in smokers.

Symptoms may include a persistent cough, coughing up blood, breathlessness, chest pains and wheezing. The earlier the cancer is diagnosed, the greater the chance of a cure through surgery, radiotherapy and/or anticancer drugs. However, less than 10 per cent of men survive for five years or more after lung cancer has been diagnosed, so prevention is crucial.

Skin cancer

In second place come the various types of skin cancer, the most common of which are squamous cell carcinoma, basal cell carcinoma and malignant melanoma. Although we know that roughly nine out of every 10 skin cancers are non-melanoma skin cancers (NMSCs), the number of new cases of these NMSCs is impossible to estimate as many remain undiagnosed. For malignant melanomas, there are over 6 cases per 100,000 men newly diagnosed in the UK each year, with an annual death rate in men of close to 2,000. The most important risk factor for skin cancer is excessive exposure to sunlight.

With the exception of malignant melanoma, most skin cancers are no threat to life or health and can usually be cured if treated early. It is essential to report any changes in your skin – such as a new lump or bump, or an alteration in the shape, size or colour of a mole – to your doctor. Treatment is usually surgical removal, sometimes followed up by radiotherapy or chemotherapy.

Large bowel cancer

The third most common type of cancer in men affects the colon or rectum. Just over 50 new cases per 100,000 men are reported in the UK each year, with an annual death rate in men of close to 16,000. This form of cancer usually develops between the ages of 50 and 70 years.

The exact cause of large bowel cancer is unknown, but genetic and dietary factors are believed to play an important part. Risk factors include: eating a high-meat, high-fat, low-fibre diet, and suffering from either ulcerative colitis or familial polyposis coli, an inherited disorder which causes hundreds of polyps (small growths) in the colon lining.

Symptoms of this particular cancer may include a prolonged change from your normal bowel habit, such as constipation or diarrhoea lasting more than ten days, blood mixed with your stools (faeces) and a sensation of not being able to empty your bowels completely.

Radiotherapy or anticancer drugs may be used to treat large bowel cancer, in addition to surgical removal of the tumour. It may be necessary for the surgeon to create a temporary or even a permanent colostomy, where the cut end of the colon is brought to the surface of the skin and the faeces empty into a bag attached to the front of the abdomen.

About half of the people who have surgery for rectal cancer survive for at least three years after the operation and 40 per cent are alive ten years later. About half of the patients who are able to have a colon cancer removed surgically survive for five years or more.

Prostate cancer

With celebrity sufferers, from Frank Zappa and Roger Moore to Norman Schwarzkopf and François Mitterrand, the media spotlight has been well and truly focused on prostate cancer over the last few years. In fact, in the minds of many, prostate disease has become synonymous with men's health in general. However, while there is no doubt that prostate cancer is a serious and relatively common condition among men, it is just one of many health problems that men in the UK have to face on a daily basis.

Fortunately, the majority of men who develop a prostate problem don't have cancer, but are actually suffering from a benign enlargement of their prostate gland, known medically as benign prostatic hyperplasia (BPH – see pages 262–5). Nevertheless, over 18,000 new cases of prostate cancer are diagnosed in the UK each year, with one man in eleven developing prostate cancer at some time during his life. The annual death rate from prostate cancer in the UK is approaching 10,000.

Prostate cancer occurs mainly in elderly men, with half of all cases occurring in men over the age of 75 years. Nearly all deaths due to prostate cancer have occurred in men aged over 65 years.

To put these figures into perspective, in the UK, prostate cancer is one of the most common types of cancer in men and the second most common cause of cancer death in men. Four times as many men die from prostate cancer as women die from cervical cancer.

Although the exact cause of prostate cancer remains unknown, several risk factors have been identified. For example, a man with an affected brother or father is eight times more likely to develop prostate cancer than a man without a similar family history. In addition, the typical UK diet – high in fat and low in green vegetables, cereals and pulses – may increase the risk.

Prostate cancer isn't just a threat to life, it may also cause distressing symptoms. For example, pressure from the tumour on the bladder and its outlet, the urethra, may cause difficulty and pain passing urine. Reassuringly, though, for many men, when urinary symptoms do occur they are due to BPH, a condition ten times more common than prostate cancer. Unfortunately, in many cases, cancer of the prostate does not produce any symptoms until it has already spread to other parts of the body. Screening for prostate cancer before it causes symptoms may be done by a simple blood test to measure the level of the protein prostate specific antigen (PSA), and by a digital rectal examination, whereby the doctor inserts a gloved, lubricated finger into the rectum to feel whether the prostate has become abnormally hard or knobbly. Additional screening tests may include an ultrasound scan.

The need for routine screening for prostate cancer remains controversial. We know from a recent Medical Research Council trial that surgical or hormonal treatment of prostate cancer that is diagnosed before it has started to cause symptoms, even though it has already spread, improves the chances of survival and reduces the incidence of severe complications. However, we do not know yet whether surgical treatment for early stage prostate cancer, detected before it causes symptoms or has spread, will have any overall benefit on survival and quality of life. The screening debate is made even more complicated by the fact that as this type of cancer is often slow-growing, many elderly men with prostate cancer will die of another cause before their cancer becomes life-threatening.

Because surgical removal of a cancerous prostate may lead to urinary incontinence and also erectile dysfunction (impotence), the specialist may decide to leave the tumour undisturbed. Radiotherapy and hormonal treatments are often used as an alternative, particularly when the cancer is already widespread when first diagnosed.

Surgical castration was occasionally carried out to slow down the progress of this disease, by removing the stimulant effect of testicular testosterone. However, advances in hormonal therapy mean that it is now possible to achieve the same result as surgical castration using regular injections of a hormone, for example goserelin ('Zoladex'), buserelin ('Suprefact'), leuprorelin ('Prostap SR') and triptorelin (Decapeptyl SR), which switch off the production of testosterone by the testicles. This so-called medical castration often results in side effects, such as hot flushes and impotence, but quality of life tends to be better in those men treated in this way.

Specialists may also prescribe a second type of drug to prostate cancer patients, known as an anti-androgen. By blocking the growth-stimulating effect of testosterone on the prostate tumour cells, anti-androgens such as 'Casodex', flutamide ('Drogenil') and cyproterone acetate ('Cyprostat') help to stop the cancer from spreading.

Male breast cancer

Although breast cancer is extremely rare in men, with less than one in every 100 cases involving a man, studies of survival following treatment of breast cancer show that these men do significantly less well than women. This is thought to be due to the fact that men delay seeking medical help, which means that their breast cancer is much more advanced when it is eventually diagnosed.

Any man noticing a lump in his breast should therefore get it checked out by a doctor as soon as possible. The earlier treatment can be started with surgical removal of the lump, followed by radiation and/or chemotherapy, the better the chance he has of surviving for at least another five or ten years.

Testicular cancer

While cancer of one of the testicles is very rare before puberty and in old age, it is actually the most common cancer in men between the ages of 15 and 49 years. In 1997 in the UK an estimated 1,500 men developed testicular cancer, and, in the same year, testicular cancer killed 90 men.

The incidence of testicular cancer has doubled since the 1970s. Although the reasons for this increase are unknown, one possible factor is the greater number of young boys suffering from an undescended testicle, which has been found to make them five times more likely to develop testicular cancer in adulthood. Corrective surgery performed on an undescended testicle before the boy reaches the age of five makes it easier to detect any subsequent formation of testicular cancer.

There may also be a hereditary factor: for example, having a brother with testicular cancer increases this cancer risk by nearly ten times.

With one type of testicular cancer – a seminoma – radiotherapy is usually given routinely after surgical removal of the affected testicle. For the other main type – a teratoma – chemotherapy may be necessary if X-rays, an ultrasound scan or blood tests show any evidence of spread.

If picked up early, over 90 per cent of testicular cancers can be cured and, providing the remaining testicle is healthy, treatment should not interfere with fertility or potency. Regular self-examination of the testicles (see page 88) is therefore essential to allow early diagnosis. It does not need to be done obsessively, but men should be aware of how their testicles normally feel so that they can spot any change in size, shape or firmness.

Coeliac disease

This rare inherited bowel disorder is caused by intolerance of a protein known as gluten, which is found in wheat, rye and other cereals. Any exposure to gluten in the diet damages the tiny projections found on the inner lining of the small intestine, interfering with the absorption of nutrients as a result.

In the UK, coeliac disease affects about 40 per 100,000 of the population. Infants with the disease will start to develop symptoms as soon as they are put on a cereal diet, with bloating of their abdomen, irritability or lethargy, pale, bulky and foul smelling bowel movements and a failure to grow normally.

In some cases, the disease may not become apparent until adulthood, in which case the bowel symptoms may be a lot milder. However, the affected person may start to lose weight and become anaemic and deficient in certain vitamins and minerals.

Diagnosis may be confirmed by taking a biopsy from the lining of the small intestine and examining the removed tissue under a microscope.

Treatment involves sticking to a life-long diet completely free of gluten, which will require you to read carefully all food labels, as cereals are used as an ingredient in many types of food, including pies, soups and sauces. The only cereals that are gluten-free are rice and maize. However, nowadays, a wide range of other gluten-free products is on sale.

Once gluten has been excluded from the diet, symptoms should clear up within weeks and the individual's weight should soon return to normal. However, vitamin and mineral supplements may need to be prescribed to correct any residual deficiencies. For more information, you can contact The Coeliac Society.*

Colds and 'flu

Colds and influenza ('flu) are viral infections which may cause a variety of familiar symptoms, including sore throat, fever, runny nose, sneezing, dry cough, aches and pains, weakness and swollen glands. The main difference between a cold and 'flu is that the latter typically makes you feel too ill to do anything other than stay in bed and lasts a few days longer. If you are old or frail, 'flu is potentially fatal.

The viruses are spread through the air in tiny droplets of mucus or saliva when an infected person coughs, sneezes or speaks. Another common way to pick up the infection is rubbing your eyes with hands that have been contaminated with the virus (for example, from a door handle).

The reason why you can suffer one cold after another is that there are more than 100 different cold viruses. Acquiring immunity to one virus will not protect you from the next type of virus that comes along. You can try to keep away from anyone who is coughing and sneezing, but unfortunately people are contagious for up to two days before their symptoms actually appear.

With both colds and 'flu, you simply need to be patient while the infection runs its course. Although there are dozens of remedies to ease the symptoms (see below), anti-viral drug treatment to speed up recovery from 'flu, using a neuraminidase inhibitor (taken by mouth or inhaler), is still under investigation in clinical trials. Antibiotics won't kill viruses, but they may be prescribed to treat or prevent any secondary bacterial infection such as sinusitis, bronchitis or pneumonia.

Most men with a cold or 'flu do not need to see their doctor. Useful self-help measures include:

- drinking plenty of fluids to help replace water lost with the increase in sweating
- aspirin or paracetamol to take away aches and pains, and to bring down a high temperature (although aspirin should *not* be given to a child under 12 years old)
- salt water or aspirin gargles to relieve a sore throat
- warm drinks containing honey and lemon to ease a sore throat and dry cough
- inhalations and decongestants to relieve a blocked-up nose (do *not* take a decongestant by mouth if you have high blood pressure, heart disease or an overactive thyroid)
- using a vaporiser or humidifier to moisten dry air, which can otherwise aggravate a cough
- taking an expectorant for a loose cough, a suppressant for a persistent dry cough
- glucose (sugar) drinks to give you energy if you don't feel like eating.

Beware of taking more than one cold remedy at a time without checking with your pharmacist. Some may contain the same ingredients, so you could risk overdosing on a drug such as paracetamol, which might be fatal.

While you have a sore throat, fever or swollen glands, it is important to avoid taking any strenuous exercise, as this will not only make the infection worse, but could lead to a dangerous complication such as inflammation of the heart muscle (myocarditis). Also, after a bad bout of 'flu, rest for at least two weeks after the symptoms have gone to allow your body to make a full recovery.

See your doctor if you develop:

- a prolonged (48 hours) or high fever (Temp>104°F/40°C)
- a cough producing coloured sputum or blood
- chest pains, facial pain or earache
- breathlessness or wheezing.

For most men, colds and 'flu are just a nuisance. However, if you are elderly or have any long-standing medical condition, particularly a heart or lung disorder, kidney disease, hormone abnormality, or any disease that requires you to take steroids or other immune system suppressants, there is a much greater risk of developing serious complications like pneumonia or heart failure.

An annual 'flu jab is therefore recommended for everyone in these high-risk categories. It is designed to provide immunity against the influenza viruses expected to be around that year. 'Flu vaccination is normally given in September or October. Do *not* wait until a 'flu epidemic has already started, as the vaccine takes up to two weeks to become effective.

Cold sores

Cold sores are painful, ugly blisters, which generally appear on the lower lip. As many as 90 per cent of the population in the UK will be exposed to the *herpes simplex* virus that causes cold sores. The initial attack, which usually occurs before the age of five years, often passes unnoticed, although some children develop flu-like symptoms, sometimes accompanied by painful ulcers on the mouth and lips.

Interestingly, most people are then immune to any further outbreak of cold sores – the virus simply lies dormant within nerve cells in their body. However, roughly one in five of those who were infected go on to suffer from recurrent cold sores.

They may strike as often as three to four times a year and nearly always involve the same part of the face. Factors that may trigger reactivation of the virus include:

- strong sunlight
- colds/feverish illness
- stress/being run down.

Most sufferers usually have warning symptoms, such as an itching, tingling, burning or prickling sensation, which may continue for 24 hours before the blisters start to appear. Typically, a cluster of small, fluid-filled blisters develops, which then breaks open to form shallow ulcers before crusting over. Apart from the lower lip, cold sores may also appear on the upper lip, corner of the mouth or just inside one of the nostrils.

If you suffer from recurrent cold sores, buy a small tube of the antiviral cream aciclovir (Zovirax) from the pharmacy or ask your GP to prescribe you a tube to keep on standby. Applied early, as soon as the warning symptoms start, Zovirax penetrates below the skin to stop the virus from multiplying. As a result, the cold sore should heal up more rapidly. If pus appears in the blisters or you develop a fever, you should see your doctor as this suggests the cold sore has become infected with bacteria.

Because cold sores contain infected material, you should also take the following precautions until the sores have healed:

- wash hands after applying the cream or accidentally touching the sores
- do not share flannels or towels
- if you wear contact lenses do not use saliva to moisten them
- avoid kissing people just in case they are not immune
- avoid oral sex as there is a slight risk of this virus leading to genital herpes

Finally, if sun exposure brings out your cold sore, put sunscreen on to the vulnerable area of skin to protect it from ultraviolet rays.

Conjunctivitis

Conjunctivitis is a common condition in which the transparent membrane that covers the white of the eye and lines the insides of the eyelids (conjunctiva) becomes inflamed.

Causes of conjunctivitis include a viral or bacterial infection, allergy (for example to pollen), irritation from exposure to a dusty or smoky atmosphere or excessive exposure to strong ultraviolet light rays (for example, skiing without protective goggles).

Conjunctivitis is the most common cause of a painful red eye. The pain is typically an irritation or itchiness, and the affected eye(s) may sting, burn or feel gritty. There may also be a thin watery discharge – clear or yellow in colour – and the eyelids may become stuck together by a yellow crust, particularly on waking after sleep.

If the cause of conjunctivitis is irritation from smoke or dust, then try using an eye bath solution from the pharmacy. If the itchiness and watering is due to allergy, then you could use one of a variety of antihistamine eye drops, also available from the pharmacy. However, if the symptoms do not settle down, or they are caused by something else, then it is important to have your eyes examined by a doctor.

Antibiotic ointment or drops will be prescribed to treat conjunctivitis caused by a bacterial infection. In addition, you may need to use warm water and disposable tissues to gently wipe away crusts from the eyelids. To prevent the infection spreading to others, avoid sharing a flannel, towel or pillowcase and put them all in the wash once the symptoms have cleared. If you wear contact lenses, they should be thoroughly cleansed and not worn again until the infection has gone.

Finally, see your doctor at once if your painful red eye is accompanied by a dull ache from within the eye, worsening pain, blurred vision or seeing coloured haloes around lights, as you may have a more serious eye condition such as glaucoma (see page 224–5).

Creutzfeld-Jakob disease (CJD)

There has been a lot of publicity, both in the newspapers and on television, about CJD since the announcement in early 1996 by the Department of Health that this previously extremely rare form of dementia had killed 10 formerly healthy young people. When the brains of these victims were examined at post-mortem, the disease appeared to have caused changes very different from the classical form of CJD, but very similar to the effects of Bovine Spongiform Encephalopathy (BSE) on the brains of cattle.

Not surprisingly, this led to this new variant of CJD (nvCJD) being called the human form of mad cow disease, and research into the link between BSE and nvCJD has intensified. Originally, government experts had thought that BSE could not be transmitted to humans. Now, they believe that the 'most likely explanation' for these cases of nvCJD was exposure to BSE before the introduction of the various precautions outlined below.

Classical CJD

The classical or sporadic form of CJD (spCJD), which affects about one person in a million in the UK (mainly elderly people) is thought to be due to infection with a 'prion' protein or a 'slow virus' – one that starts to cause signs of disease only months or years after the original infection.

In addition to a progressive deterioration in intellectual function and personality, the victim develops sudden muscle contractions and loses the ability to co-ordinate movements. In an advanced stage of the disease, the person may go blind and be unable to speak. There is no cure, and death usually occurs within 12 months.

nvCJD

The symptoms of nvCJD are similar to those of spCJD but usually begin with unsteadiness when walking and a difficulty with speech before dementia becomes apparent. There is no cure as yet, and death usually occurs within two years.

Although the exact cause of this new form of CJD is unknown, the victims (27 in total at the time of writing) are thought to have been exposed to the same disease agent as BSE through eating infected beef before the various measures to minimise this risk had come into effect. However, whether this nvCJD/BSE agent is a 'prion' protein or a 'slow virus' remains unknown.

With the ban on feeding cattle with meat and bone meal from any farm animal, the compulsory slaughter of cattle thought to be already infected with BSE, the removal of brain, spinal cord, retinas and offal from animals that have been slaughtered for food, and a ban on the consumption of beef on the bone and the use of beef bones in stock cubes, it is hoped that an epidemic of nvCJD can be prevented.

Although there are no cases in which nvCJD has been shown to have arisen from blood or blood products, as a precautionary measure, supplies of factor VIII for haemophiliacs, immunoglobulin used in tetanus vaccine and human albumin used to stabilise many vaccines are no longer being used when they have been extracted from UK donors. In addition, the government announced in July 1998 that it would be introducing a procedure known as leucodepletion – the removal of white blood cells – to reduce any theoretical risk of donated blood being contaminated.

With the recent discovery of nvCJD in the appendix of a patient who later developed the disease, research is now underway to test anonymously several thousand specimens kept from previous appendix removals to establish how many other people in the population might be expected to develop nvCJD.

For more information on CJD, or to talk to others who have looked after someone with this condition, you should contact the National CJD Support Network* or the Human BSE Foundation.*

Crohn's disease

Crohn's disease is a long-term condition in which the inner lining of parts of the small and/or large bowel become inflamed. Although it may develop at any age, Crohn's disease usually starts in early adulthood. In the UK as many as 4,000 new cases are diagnosed each year, and the incidence is on the increase.

Although the cause of the bowel inflammation is still unknown, it is thought that a genetic susceptibility and specific environmental factors both play a role. Factors that have been implicated, but not proven, include:

- intolerance to certain foods
- the measles virus
- the measles vaccine
- bacteria known as Mycobacterium paratuberculosis, which cause a condition very similar to Crohn's disease in cattle and sheep.

Symptoms of Crohn's disease, which tend to fluctuate in severity, include diarrhoea, abdominal pain and cramps, blood mixed with the faeces, fever and weight loss. Because the inflammation can also affect other parts of the digestive tract, sores may appear in the mouth and around the anus. Inflammation may also occur elsewhere in the body, for example, causing joint pains and irritation of the skin and eyes.

Diagnosis can be confirmed using an endoscope (fibre-optic telescope that is passed up through the anus into the large bowel) and/or barium X-rays, which show up the areas of inflammation and ulceration in the bowel lining.

Treatment to control the inflammation may include corticosteroids given by mouth and sometimes as an enema; sulphasalazine; and other more powerful drugs which suppress the body's natural immune system. Surgery may be needed if the inflammation has resulted in loops of bowel becoming obstructed, if abnormal channels (fistula) have developed between loops of bowel or if abscesses have formed.

During an acute flare up, some specialists recommend the so-called spaceman's diet: liquid food which is completely absorbed before it reaches the end of the small bowel (useful when you are weightless inside a space capsule), thereby resting the inflamed bowel wall.

Eventually the disease may burn itself out, although most sufferers need to continue with medication and stick to a bland diet that is low in high-fibre foods to keep their symptoms under reasonable control. Crohn's disease does not increase the risk of bowel cancer.

For more information, you should contact the National Association for Colitis and Crohn's disease.*

Dandruff

There is no need to be embarrassed if you suffer from dandruff. It is an extremely common problem which affects nearly half the population of the UK at some time in their lives. Dandruff is harmless and, most important of all, it is easy to treat.

The unsightly white flakes that appear in your hair and on the collar and shoulders of your clothes are actually clumps of dead skin cells which are being continuously shed from your scalp. Like the skin over the rest of your body, your scalp has a protective outer layer of dead cells which loosen and drop off, to be replaced by new cells moving up from the deeper layers. Normally, these skin scales are too small and too few to be noticed. It is when they clump together and start to flake off in much greater numbers that they become visible. Although excessive skin flaking can happen on any part of your body, it most commonly affects the scalp in the form of dandruff. If this condition does spread to other areas, usually the eyebrows, around the nose and the front of the chest, it is called seborrhoeic dermatitis.

Mild dandruff may be treated with a medicated shampoo bought from a pharmacist. This type of shampoo contains a substance (selenium) which penetrates into the scalp and slows down the over-production of skin cells.

If your dandruff is accompanied by an itchy, inflamed rash on your scalp, make an appointment to see your doctor. You may need to be prescribed a corticosteroid cream or lotion to ease the inflammation.

In many cases, persistent dandruff and seborrhoeic dermatitis are the result of a yeast infection and the only effective remedy is an antifungal drug, prescribed as a shampoo for the scalp and a cream to apply to any other affected areas of your skin. Treatment normally has to be continued for at least one month and some people need to go on using the shampoo on a regular basis to stop the dandruff coming back.

Deafness

Deafness is perceived as a serious handicap because it acts as a barrier to normal conversation, encouraging the sufferer to become increasingly isolated and depressed as a result. In children, deafness can interfere with learning and speech development.

In conductive deafness there is something interfering with the normal transmission of sound waves through the ear canal, the middle ear and into the inner ear. Sensorineural deafness is caused by damage to the hearing mechanism in the inner ear, or to the acoustic nerve that carries sound impulses from the inner ear to the brain.

In adults, the most common reason for conductive deafness is a build-up of earwax; simply using eardrops and having the ear canals syringed with warm water by a doctor can restore hearing to a satisfactory level. A perforated eardrum can also result in conductive deafness; if this injury doesn't heal within two months, it may need to be repaired surgically. Another cause is otosclerosis, where one of the tiny connecting bones inside the middle ear – the stapes – becomes immobile. To correct this form of deafness, the rigid stapes bone may be removed and an artificial replacement inserted.

Sensorineural deafness may be brought on as a result of prolonged exposure to loud noise, by a viral infection such as meningitis, or as a toxic reaction to certain medications.

If you are having trouble with your hearing, the first step is to overcome any embarrassment and discuss the problem with your doctor so that any treatable cause can be dealt with. Your GP may refer you to an ear, nose and throat (ENT) clinic or hearing-aid centre for a full assessment of your hearing and to see whether a hearing aid might help. However, be warned that in some parts of the UK there are long waiting lists for this service on the NHS. Also, however sophisticated the hearing aid, it will only be able to amplify those sound frequencies you have difficulty detecting; it will not give you back perfect hearing.

A new treatment for complete sensorineural deafness, that has only been available in recent years, involves the insertion of a cochlear implant – an electronic device which can detect sound waves and transmit them to the brain. As a result of further refinements in the technology, a small number of people have had reasonable hearing restored with this device.

Dementia

Dementia is a deterioration in mental ability characterised by loss of short-term memory, impairment of intellect, disorientation and confusion. Although dementia is more common in elderly people, it is not confined to this age group and is not an inevitable part of growing old.

About one in 10 men over the age of 65, and one in five over the age of 75, have some degree of dementia. However, in most cases, this consists only of occasional absentmindedness and does not interfere with the man's ability to lead a normal life.

The most common cause of dementia is Alzheimer's disease (see pages 186–7). Another frequent cause is narrowing and hardening of the arteries in the brain. Dementia may also develop as a result of a head injury, brain infection, brain tumour, alcoholism, drug abuse, underactive thyroid or deficiency of vitamin B_{12}. Symptoms may come on gradually over several years.

The doctor may carry out a physical examination and blood tests to establish if the cause is treatable. Most men suffering from mild dementia can lead a near-normal life, although it is important for them to have some form of regular supervision, even if it is just a brief daily visit. In more severe cases, constant supervision may be required as the individual may be at risk of harming himself or others.

Depression

Everyone complains of being depressed occasionally, by which they mean feeling miserable, fed-up or pessimistic, as a result of a disappointment or frustration in their life. Depression becomes an illness that needs medical attention or psychological treatment when it persists, deepens or starts to dominate an individual's existence.

This severe form of depression is typified by a loss of interest and enjoyment in life, feelings of helplessness or inadequacy and a lack of drive and motivation. The sufferer may start to have difficulty in making decisions and may no longer be able to cope at work; personal relationships with friends and family may be put under strain. He may begin to feel that life is no longer worth living.

About one in every nine men visits his family doctor because of a serious episode of depression. In some cases, there may be an obvious cause such as divorce or another relationship problem, unemployment, physical illness or money worries. However, depression may hit others completely out of the blue, which makes it more difficult for their friends and family to be supportive. One common type of depression, known as seasonal affective disorder (see pages 271), is thought to be due to a chemical change in the brain brought on by a lack of exposure to ultraviolet light during the winter months.

Warning symptoms of depression that may need to be treated if they persist include:

- insomnia and regular waking in the early hours of the morning
- generalised aches and pains
- sense of despair
- difficulty concentrating on one task
- marked increase or decrease in appetite
- reduced sex drive
- loss of self-confidence
- crying for no apparent reason.

Confusion, agitation, extreme apathy and drinking more alcohol than usual can all be triggered by depression. Often a friend or relative has to persuade the depressed person to go to the doctor. Any threat of 'ending it all' should be taken seriously and the doctor called out if necessary.

SELF-HELP MEASURES TO TREAT OR PREVENT DEPRESSION

- talk problems and worries through with a friend or relative
- don't bottle up your emotions – it can help to re-live painful experiences and to cry if you want to
- take some form of regular physical activity
- eat a healthy, balanced diet even when you don't feel hungry
- don't drink alcohol to feel better – the immediate relief will only be followed by a deeper depression
- if the thought of retirement is at the root of your problem, make positive plans to stay mentally and physically active.

However, do not delay seeking medical advice if these measures do not help you.

A few people suffering from severe depression also occasionally feel elated and overactive at times. This condition is known as manic depression and is typically treated with a drug called lithium.

A serious bout of depression should not be allowed to continue without treatment and will usually not disappear on its own. The risk of suicide is greatest among elderly men who have become isolated, or who are suffering from a long-term or painful illness, but the numbers of suicides in younger men is on the increase, typically involving a violent method such as hanging.

Treatment of depression, which is usually highly effective, may consist of:

- psychotherapy (see Glossary) or counselling from a trained professional who will encourage the depressed individual to talk about his feelings and to explore and confront the possible reasons for them
- antidepressants, which normally take a few weeks to lift the depression but can improve any associated anxiety or sleeping difficulties more rapidly. Unlike tranquillisers, antidepressants are not addictive. Treatment will invariably be continued for several months after the symptoms have gone to reduce the chance of a relapse

- electroconvulsive therapy (ECT), reserved for severe depression that is either not responding to other treatment or is accompanied by delusions. An electric current is passed through the brain for a split second with the patient under a light general anaesthetic.

Diabetes

Diabetes mellitus (sugar diabetes) is a common disorder of the body's metabolism in which the pancreas gland either ceases to produce, or produces very much less of the hormone insulin. Insulin is responsible for the absorption of glucose (sugar) from the bloodstream into the body's cells, where it is converted into energy. Another important function of insulin is to control the uptake of glucose into the liver and muscle cells, where it is stored as glycogen (starch).

Symptoms occur partly due to an abnormally high concentration of glucose building up in the blood and partly to the body's inability to use or store glucose properly. Also, fat metabolism will be disrupted, resulting in an increase in blood cholesterol, which in turn increases the risk of a heart attack or stroke.

WARNING SYMPTOMS OF DIABETES

- blurred vision
- excessive thirst
- frequent urination
- fatigue and weakness
- numbness and tingling in the feet and hands.

There are two main types of diabetes: insulin-dependent, also known as juvenile-onset or Type 1 diabetes, and non-insulin-dependent, often referred to as maturity-onset or Type 2. Insulin-dependent diabetes is the more severe form, which usually appears suddenly at some time before the age of 35. Destruction of the insulin-producing cells in the pancreas leads to complete or almost complete absence of insulin, which must be replaced by daily injections of an insulin substitute, either synthetic or from an animal. Cell destruction in the pancreas is thought to be due to an abnormal immune response to a viral infection, or to some unknown environmental factor in those people who are genetically predisposed to this disease, but the cause is still under investigation.

In non-insulin-dependent diabetes, which usually comes on gradually after the age of 40, some insulin is still being produced but not enough to meet the body's needs. There is a strong genetic predisposition to this form of diabetes; however, ageing and obesity also play a key role in provoking its onset: as you get older, the pancreas begins to function less efficiently and excess body fat hinders the use of available insulin.

Whereas insulin-dependent diabetes usually causes obvious symptoms, many people with the non-insulin-dependent type only become aware of it as the result of a routine blood or urine test, which reveals abnormally high levels of blood sugar, or the presence of sugar in the urine.

SELF-HELP MEASURES TO ASSIST YOUR TREATMENT

- eat fewer refined carbohydrate (sugary) foods and more high-fibre, unrefined carbohydrate (starchy) foods, to avoid marked fluctuations in blood glucose levels
- cut down on fatty foods, particularly saturated fats
- lose any excess weight through regular exercise and the above diet
- get into a medication routine to reduce the chance of missing a dose
- carefully monitor either your blood or urine glucose
- have regular diabetic check-ups with a specialist in diabetes (this may be your GP or at a hospital clinic)
- carry or wear at all times a card identifying you as a diabetic in the event of an emergency
- be aware of the warning symptoms of hypoglycaemia (a dangerously low blood sugar level), which include feeling dizzy or drowsy, sweating, tingling, cold clammy skin, palpitations and headache. If such symptoms occur, a sugary drink or food should be taken at once to prevent collapse and coma.
- be aware also of the symptoms of hyperglycaemia (acetone odour on the breath, drowsiness, confusion and, in severe cases, lapsing into a coma), in which the blood sugar level becomes dangerously high. This may be caused by eating too many sugary foods and/or not taking enough medication.

The aim of treatment is to keep the blood glucose level as near normal as possible by keeping food and insulin intake well balanced. While insulin-dependent diabetics require insulin injections to achieve this, most non-insulin-dependent diabetics control their condition by means of a specific diet and/or antidiabetic tablets; the latter work either by stimulating the pancreas to produce more insulin or by making cells more sensitive to the action of insulin.

With proper treatment and monitoring, the risk of complications, such as damage to the eyes, nerves, blood vessels and kidneys, can be reduced and most diabetics are able to lead a full and active life.

Diarrhoea

Diarrhoea is an increased frequency of bowel movements above what is normal for that individual, along with the passage of loose, watery stools. The numerous different causes of diarrhoea, include:

- irritation of the bowel lining by rich or spicy foods
- drinking large amounts of alcohol
- antibiotic side-effect due to the eradication of friendly bacteria in the bowel
- food poisoning (see pages 225–6)
- viral gastroenteritis/gastric flu
- traveller's diarrhoea due to exposure to new types of bacteria in foreign food and drink
- irritable bowel syndrome (see pages 241–2)
- food allergy (usually with other symptoms such as a skin rash)
- Crohn's disease (see pages 212–13)
- ulcerative colitis
- overactive thyroid
- bowel cancer (rare cause).

Most cases of diarrhoea clear up within a few days. Drugs to stop diarrhoea are best avoided unless you need to travel somewhere or you have to work that day. This is because if the cause is an infection, diarrhoea is the body's natural way of expelling the bugs. Also, if you take several doses, you might prolong the illness or end up with rebound constipation.

The best treatment is an oral rehydration therapy from the pharmacy, which contains glucose for energy and replaces not just fluid but also the potassium and sodium salts which are lost from the body.

You can make your own solution by adding eight level teaspoons of sugar and one level teaspoon of salt for each litre of water – but be careful to get these measures right as too much salt can cause vomiting, which will make you more dehydrated.

Additional drinks may include flat lemonade or flat cola, but avoid milk, coffee and strong tea. Once the diarrhoea has stopped for 24 hours, you can start eating solid food again, beginning with starchy products such as bread, toast and cereals, and lean meats such as chicken. It is best to keep your intake of fat to a minimum for a few days, for example switch to skimmed milk, as if the bowel is still inflamed, too much fat may cause the diarrhoea to return.

If diarrhoea persists for over 48 hours, or for more than 24 hours in a very young or elderly person, then see the doctor. You should also seek medical attention if there are other symptoms, such as blood or mucus in the stools or a high fever or headache, if signs of dehydration appear such as dry mouth, sunken eyes and drowsiness or if you have recurrent attacks of diarrhoea.

Epilepsy

Epilepsy is a brain disorder in which there is a tendency to suffer recurrent seizures due to a disturbance in the brain's electrical activity. Normally, brain cells send impulses to each other and to other nerve cells in an organised, controlled manner. During an epileptic seizure, however, this well-ordered system breaks down, with impulses emitted simultaneously, continuously and rapidly. Seizure intensity may vary between violent convulsions with prolonged loss of consciousness to brief lapses in concentration.

About one in 200 men suffer from epilepsy at some time in their lives, with almost three-quarters being diagnosed before the age of 20. However, having a seizure does not mean the onset of epilepsy; many of the people who do not have a recurrence within a few weeks never have another attack. In many men, epilepsy may develop for no obvious reason, but possible causes include alcohol or drug withdrawal, damage to the brain from a head injury, stroke, tumour or infection.

The doctor will begin by asking for a description of the type of seizure from someone who has witnessed an attack. Epileptic seizures may be divided into either generalised or partial depending on the part of the brain affected. While generalised seizures affect the entire brain

---

FIRST-AID TREATMENT FOR A SEIZURE

- stop others crowding around
- place something soft under the head
- carefully loosen clothing around the neck
- do not restrain the person
- do not put anything into the mouth
- do not try to move him unless he is in danger where he is
- once the seizure is over roll him on to his side and check nothing is blocking his airway
- seek medical help if the seizure continues for longer than five minutes, another seizure immediately follows the first or if the person remains unconscious.

---

area, partial seizures affect specific regions. Partial seizures can in turn be divided into two types: simple partial, where patients display convulsions but remain aware of their surroundings, and complex partial, where the sufferer's consciousness is affected either at the beginning or during the seizure.

Many men who suffer from epilepsy lead normal lives, with no symptoms between attacks. Some experience warning symptoms before a seizure, in the form of an 'aura', for example feeling odd, restless or uncomfortable.

Diagnostic tests may include an electroencephalogram (EEG) to measure electrical activity in the brain, along with imaging procedures such as a CT or MRI scan to show the brain structure in detail. Blood tests may also be carried out to check for signs of kidney or liver failure, which may also cause recurrent seizures.

To bring seizures under control, the doctor may prescribe one or a combination of anti-epileptic drugs. These work either by blocking the action of excitatory brain chemicals or by increasing the action of inhibitory brain chemicals.

In addition to taking this medication reliably, anyone suffering from epilepsy should try to avoid any circumstance likely to provoke a seizure, such as:

- extreme tiredness
- dehydration

- not eating properly
- flashing lights (in anyone with 'photosensitive epilepsy').

Once a man has been diagnosed as suffering from epilepsy, he will have to inform the DVLA and will not be allowed to drive until either he has been seizure-free for one year or the seizures have been only at night for three years.

Finally, about one-third of men with epilepsy eventually stop having seizures. The doctor may therefore gradually withdraw anti-epileptic treatment if no seizure has occurred for over three years. For more information, contact the British Epilepsy Association.*

Eye and vision problems

The most common reason for someone's vision becoming blurred is a problem with the focusing mechanism in the eyes. In young men, this is usually due to myopia (short-sightedness), a condition in which the eyeball has grown too long from the front to the back. As a result, light rays from objects in the distance are focused by the cornea and lens in front of, rather than directly on to, the retina. While close vision remains unaffected, anything more than a few yards away will no longer appear sharply defined: for example, there may be difficulty in recognising people at a distance.

For most men, myopia comes on so slowly that it is not picked up until a man has a routine eye test (see pages 90–1). An optician can then correct the defect with spectacles or contact lenses.

In a man over the age of 45, his near vision is most likely to fail due to the common eye disorder presbyobia. A weakness develops in the muscles that change the shape of the lens in each eye. As a result, it becomes more difficult for the man to focus on small print and close objects. A man who has been wearing spectacles for short-sightedness will typically find that he has to take them off when he tries to read something.

To correct presbyopia, the optician can prescribe spectacles which, if the man is also short-sighted, can be fitted with bifocal lenses – one half designed for near vision, the other for distance vision. Because the focusing power of the eye characteristically continues to weaken as a normal part of ageing, stronger lenses may be required every year or two until all the focusing is being done by the spectacles; wearing spectacles will not itself make the eye muscles weaker.

Another common focusing problem is hypermetropia (far-sightedness). In this case, because the eyeball is too short, the light rays tend to be focused behind the retina. In young men, the muscles that change the shape of the lens to boost focusing power can usually compensate for this underlying abnormality. However, as the lens muscles weaken with age, hypermetropia may start to cause blurring of close objects, and even affect distance vision in more severe cases. Spectacles or contact lenses of the correct strength should immediately restore clear vision.

In astigmatism, the front surface of the eye loses its smooth, even curve and magnification in one plane is not the same as in another. Most people's eyes have a minor degree of astigmatism which does not need to be corrected with spectacles or contact lenses.

Any disturbance in your vision should always be checked out by an optician or doctor. Many different disorders can interfere with normal vision: most involve a particular structure in one or both eyes, but a few are the result of interference to the passage of nerve impulses from the retina to the brain, or damage to the area of the brain where pictures are received and interpreted.

Common eye disorders not corrected with lenses
Cataract

A cataract is a loss of transparency in the lens of one or both eyes, causing vision to become increasingly blurred, with red, orange and yellow colours becoming more pronounced than others. The risk of developing a cataract increases with age; in young men, there is usually a specific reason for this change: diabetes or a serious eye injury, for example. Surgical removal of the opaque lens and replacement with a tiny artificial lens implant usually restores normal vision.

Glaucoma

Glaucoma, in which abnormally high pressure inside one or both eyes interferes with the blood supply to the nerve at the back of the affected eye(s), may cause permanent blindness. In some cases there are obvious symptoms – a painful red eye with blurred vision, or seeing coloured haloes around lights, for example. However, it is often only picked up during a routine eye examination if an optician or doctor carries out a pressure test. Because glaucoma runs in families, anyone who has a close relative with this disorder needs regular screening after the age of 40.

Treatment of glaucoma is with daily application of pressure-reducing eye drops and, sometimes, drainage surgery. Vision cannot be restored, but further deterioration can be prevented.

Retinal detachment

Separation of the retina from the outer layers at the back of the eye sometimes follows a blow to the eye, but, more usually, occurs spontaneously due to natural degeneration. Detachment is more common in men who are extremely short-sighted.

A retinal detachment may develop without any warning symptoms, with the man suddenly noticing a 'black curtain', which has obscured his vision in the affected eye. However, there will often be a burst of flashing lights as the tear stimulates the light-sensitive nerve cells in the retina, accompanied by the appearance of spots in front of the eye.

Surgical treatment of a retinal detachment usually achieves excellent results, as long as the operation is performed before the damage has spread to the central part of the retina (macula), an area densely packed with light receptors, which assists the perception of fine detail.

Food poisoning

Food poisoning is an illness brought on by eating food or drinking water that is contaminated with bacteria, viruses, worms, chemicals or toxins. Symptoms usually consist of abdominal cramps, nausea, vomiting and diarrhoea, although some types of food poisoning may result in headaches, fever, rash or muscle pains. Listeriosis, for example, typically causes 'flu-like symptoms without ever upsetting the stomach.

The symptoms of food poisoning usually come on suddenly, within about 48 hours of consuming contaminated food or drink. However, because this time can vary from as short as 30 minutes to as long as 30 days, depending on the bug or chemical involved, you should not automatically blame the last thing you ate or drank. Food poisoning is usually suspected if several people become ill after eating the same food.

The number of cases of food poisoning reported by doctors in the UK over the last few years has increased massively. However, because most people do not go to their doctor for treatment, the true incidence is thought to be even higher, with as many as half a million cases each year in the UK.

No food or drink is completely sterile. It all contains small amounts of a variety of bugs. However, most of these bugs are harmless and are destroyed by stomach acids. Bugs in food and drink tend to cause problems only if there are large numbers of them or if a particular type such as salmonella is present.

Farm animals, especially poultry, often harbour salmonella, which is why frozen meat must always be thawed sufficiently to allow it to be cooked properly. The most common causes of food poisoning are the result of basic mistakes in the kitchen, such as allowing raw meat to come into contact with cooked meat or not re-heating a meat dish for long enough in the microwave. Because salmonella is found in some eggs, it is advisable not to eat them lightly cooked or raw (as in mayonnaise).

It is also important to wash carefully any fruit, vegetable or salad, even if it looks clean, to remove listeria, a bacteria commonly found in vegetation and soil. One major reason for the apparent epidemic in food poisoning is the increase in consumption of convenience foods, such as pre-packed salads. Food that is not freshly prepared and eaten the same day is much more likely to contain larger numbers of bugs.

If you visit any country where tap water is unclean, you should avoid salads and raw vegetables, only eat fruit that can be peeled and do not have ice-cream or ice in your drinks. Also, you should drink only bottled water and use it to clean your teeth.

An attack of food poisoning is not usually serious. The symptoms disappear as quickly and dramatically as they came on, normally within a few days. Treatment of diarrhoea caused by food poisoning is discussed in detail on pages 220–21. The source of contaminated food or drink will be suggested by the types of food you have been eating and how long it took for the symptoms to come on. Certain types of bug are found more commonly in particular foods, and each has its own characteristic incubation period. Tests to confirm the cause may involve sending samples of vomit, faeces or any suspect leftover food to the laboratory for analysis.

Gallstones

Gallstones are crystals of cholesterol, calcium and/or bile pigment that form inside the gallbladder. These stones may be as small as grains of sand or as large as walnuts. The gall bladder is a sac-like organ located under the liver, which stores bile produced from the liver and passes it on to the duodenum, where it helps in the digestion of fatty food.

The formation of gallstones is thought to be due to an imbalance in the different chemicals that make up bile. Excess cholesterol in the bile from eating too much fatty food may be a contributory factor. Gallstones are more common in elderly and overweight people.

Gallstones may be picked up on a routine X-ray; in which case, if they are not causing any symptoms, they can be left untreated. However, in some people, gallstones cause intermittent attacks of colicky abdominal pain, usually on the right side of the upper part of the abdomen, typically brought on by eating fatty foods, and sometimes spreading through to the back and under the right shoulder blade. Other symptoms during an attack of 'biliary colic' may include fever, chills, nausea, vomiting and jaundice.

Diagnosis can usually be confirmed from an ultrasound scan. Drug treatment to dissolve the stones may be tried, but this can take several months, and new stones often form after medication is stopped. Surgical removal of the gallbladder is usually advised if the stones are causing recurrent attacks of pain or other complications, such as cholecystitis or pancreatitis, occur. A few people find that fatty foods continue to disagree with them after the operation, but there are usually no after-effects. New surgical techniques to remove gallstones include:

- the use of shock waves to shatter the stones into powder
- key-hole surgery, where the gallbladder is removed using instruments passed into the abdomen through a fibre-optic telescope, thus avoiding the need for the surgeon to make a long incision.

German measles

German measles (rubella) is a viral infection that occurs most commonly among children between the ages of six and 12. Despite its name, German measles is similar to measles only in that both these illnesses cause a pink spotted rash. Whereas measles can make a child extremely unwell for a few days and is often associated with complications such as middle ear infection and pneumonia, German measles usually only causes mild symptoms, such as:

- slight fever
- rash of small, flat pink spots, which usually begins on the face and spreads down the neck on to the chest, abdomen, back and limbs, disappearing after a few days
- enlarged lymph glands at the back of the neck
- joint pains after the rash has faded.

These symptoms are easily confused with those of other conditions, such as other types of viral infection or a food allergy. In adolescents and adults, the symptoms may be more troublesome and are more likely to include headache.

The German measles virus is spread in droplets, for example during coughing and sneezing. Symptoms typically first appear after an incubation period of between 14 and 21 days. An individual may be infectious from a few days before his symptoms appear until one day after they clear up.

Although German measles was once a common childhood infection, in the UK it is now relatively rare due to its inclusion in the routine immunisation programme. Immunisation against German measles was introduced to reduce the risk of pregnant women being exposed to this infection. Contracted during the first four months of pregnancy, the German measles virus can pass to the foetus through the placenta and cause miscarriage and serious birth defects.

Glandular fever

Glandular fever, also known as infectious mononucleosis, is a viral infection which most commonly affects adolescents and young adults. It is sometimes called the 'kissing disease' because the virus may be carried in saliva exchanged during a wet mouth-to-mouth kiss.

Routine blood testing suggests that as many as 50 per cent of the population in the UK may have been infected with this virus. Only a small number of these people will actually develop symptoms, but all of them will continue to release the active virus into their saliva intermittently for the rest of their lives. Infection with glandular fever is most likely to be picked up from close contact with one of these symptom-free carriers, rather than someone who is obviously ill.

Typically, glandular fever starts with 'flu-like symptoms - sore throat, high temperature, headache, weakness, aches and pains - and soon afterwards lymph nodes in the neck, armpits and groin become swollen and tender. A blood test which shows the presence of abnormal antibodies in the circulation will confirm the diagnosis. However, some people suffering from a glandular fever-like illness have a negative blood test at first that only becomes positive after a few weeks.

Because it is caused by a virus, antibiotics will not cure glandular fever. The only treatment is rest and relaxation while the infection runs its own course. Trying to do too much too soon will increase the chance of a relapse. Glandular fever is not usually a dangerous infection, but it can be extremely debilitating and may last for many months. The individual may suffer recurrent episodes of relapse, during which he will be unable to cope with vigorous physical or mental activity.

One possible complication is liver inflammation (hepatitis) resulting in jaundice. In most cases, normal liver function returns within a few months.

Gout

Gout is a type of arthritis that characteristically attacks one joint at a time. The joint at the base of the big toe is the one most often affected. It develops when uric acid crystals are deposited inside a joint, which cause the affected tissues to become temporarily inflamed. During an attack, the joint becomes extremely painful and swollen, with redness of the overlying skin. Occasionally, uric acid crystallises as white deposits under the skin (tophi), which may then ulcerate and have to be removed surgically.

Men are ten times more likely to suffer from attacks of gout than women, possibly due to their higher consumption of alcohol, particularly beer, and possibly due to sex differences in protein metabolism. Attacks may begin any time after puberty in men, while women usually develop this condition only after the menopause.

An attack may be treated with large doses of an anti-inflammatory drug and sometimes with the drug colchicine to suppress the inflammation rapidly. If the cause is abnormally high levels of uric acid in the blood and attacks are recurrent, the doctor may prescribe a drug which reduces the production of uric acid in the body, or a drug to increase the amount of uric acid passed in the urine.

Gout sufferers are advised to reduce their dietary intake of purine, which is converted in the body to uric acid. Foods to avoid because they are high in purine include organ meats (liver, kidney, heart), wild game, anchovies, mackerel, herring, scallops, sardines, whitebait and mussels. Foods to eat in moderation because they contain a fair amount of purine include other meats, poultry, fish not mentioned above, peas, green beans, lentils, spinach, mushrooms, asparagus and cauliflower.

Hair loss

There is no need to be alarmed when you find hairs caught in your brush or comb, or blocking the plughole after you wash your hair or take a shower. Everyone loses on average between 50 and 150 hairs each day. However, for each hair that drops out, a new hair from the same follicle normally grows up to replace it within three months.

The hair that drops out is in the resting phase of its growth cycle. At any one time, about 10 per cent of scalp hair is in this resting phase, while the remaining 90 per cent is actively growing. Loss of hair is only considered to be a problem when it starts to produce bald patches and, even then, for most men baldness results from their genetic make-up rather than from any scalp or hair disease.

Hair loss in men is most commonly due to the hereditary condition known as male-pattern baldness, in which the hair first starts to thin out over the temples and crown to cause a receding hair line. Normal hair at these sites is replaced by fine, downy hair, which eventually disappears altogether to create a slowly expanding bald area.

A few men who complain of going bald have developed one or more small, circular areas of baldness, where the exposed scalp looks and feels perfectly healthy. This condition, known as alopecia areata, remains a mystery to doctors. The cause is unknown and there is no consistently reliable treatment as yet, although, fortunately, the hair usually grows back within a few months.

Another common reason for bald patches is mistreating hair, for example, by brushing or combing it over-enthusiastically, pulling on it as a nervous habit, or adopting a hairstyle where the roots are under constant tension, for example, by pulling it into too tight a ponytail. It is also best always to use a soft-bristled brush to reduce the amount of trauma to your hair roots.

Occasionally, bald patches are due to a fungal infection, or some other skin disease affecting the scalp. In this case, the scalp will look unhealthy, there will usually be stubble rather than smooth skin and your doctor should be able to return your hair to normal by treating your scalp problem with, for example, an antifungal drug.

Factors which can cause sudden generalised loss of hair include severe stress, prolonged illness, a major operation, a crash diet and exposure to radiation. Once the individual starts to make a recovery, the hair will normally regrow within a few months. Temporary baldness may also be brought on by a number of popular medications including certain betablocker drugs, arthritis drugs and some of the drugs used to lower blood cholesterol.

There is also a rare inherited condition which, in addition to causing total baldness, results in a complete loss of body hair so that even the eyebrows and eyelashes disappear.

Whereas in the past, 'treatment' of baldness consisted of being fitted with a wig or toupée, nowadays a number of other measures are available:

- a new prescription drug to treat hair loss, known as finasteride (Propecia), which is taken as a tablet once daily. Clinical trials have shown that Propecia stimulates regrowth of hair and prevents further hair loss in 86 per cent of men with mild to moderate male-pattern baldness. One disadvantage, though, is that Propecia, having passed from the circulation into the semen, could damage an already developing foetus, so any man taking this treatment must wear a condom during sex with a female partner (who is or may become pregnant)
- a hair-restoring solution, developed from the blood pressure drug minoxidil, which can halt the progression of hair loss and stimulate some hair regrowth. However, it only seems to help some of the men who suffer from male-pattern baldness, and the hair that grows back tends to look rather fluffy. Stopping minoxidil leads to gradual loss of any hair that has been gained within four to six months and so treatment has to be continued indefinitely. Minoxidil can now be bought over the counter at the pharmacy, with one month's supply costing about £25.
- a much more expensive option which is sometimes successful in covering up a bald patch is a hair transplant. Many factors influence whether such a procedure would work well, for example, the pattern and extent of hair loss, the texture of the hair and how curvy or wavy it is. Plugs or strips of skin are transferred from hair-bearing scalp to slits or holes made in a bald or thinning area and held in

position under pressure. Sometimes, a small flap of scalp is removed as a separate procedure prior to transplantation to reduce the area needing a hair graft.

Hair transplantation usually takes three to four sessions, with four months between each, at a cost of several thousand pounds. The procedure is not available on the NHS. It is important to be patient after a hair transplant, as grafted hair is usually shed, taking several months to start growing again and growing only very slowly at first. To avoid this problem of hair fallout and delayed regrowth, it is occasionally possible to cut a flap of scalp hair which is then repositioned across a cut section of bald scalp, leaving the blood supply to the graft intact.

- hair weaving and fusion techniques have also advanced considerably over recent years. However, even the more expensive synthetic hairpieces only last for about three years.

To cope with hair loss:
- try thickening shampoos and conditioners, which either coat the hair shafts or swell individual hairs. They can help conceal an area of thinning, but there is no shampoo or over-the-counter remedy that reverses baldness
- pat rather than rub your hair dry
- while your hair is still damp, try a different parting to give it more lift
- use a spray, mousse or gel to make your hair look fuller; however, overuse of these products may cause hair to become brittle, encouraging further hair loss
- avoid long hair at the back and sides if you are thinning on top as this will highlight the bald area by pulling hair away from it
- consider having a gentle perm to disguise thinning hair by making it lift and appear fuller
- if you wear a wig or hairpiece, ask your hairdresser to style it to create a more natural look.

Hay fever

Hay fever is an allergic reaction to pollen from trees, grasses or weeds, or to spores released from fungi or moulds. Symptoms of hay fever include sneezing, a runny nose, itchy watering eyes and occasionally wheezing. The proper medical name for this condition is seasonal allergic rhinitis.

Self-help measures to prevent or reduce the symptoms of hay fever include:

- staying indoors in the early morning (before 10am) when pollen counts are usually at their highest (if possible)
- having the grass around your home mown regularly by someone other than yourself
- wearing a protective mask if you have to go outdoors when pollen levels are high
- keeping windows closed, particularly at night
- driving an air-conditioned car so that you can keep the windows and vents to the outside shut
- using a tumble dryer: pollen collects on clothes hung outdoors to dry
- asking your pharmacist to recommend an antihistamine medication, preferably one that doesn't cause dizziness or drowsiness.

See a doctor if your symptoms are severe or are making your life miserable. You should also seek medical help if you develop symptoms of allergic asthma such as a dry cough, wheezing or breathlessness.

In addition to an antihistamine drug, you may be prescribed eye drops, a nasal spray, or an inhaler to widen your airways, depending on your symptoms. A course of desensitisation injections may be successful in those people who are allergic to just one or two particular substances.

Heart attack

A heart attack, also known as a coronary thrombosis or myocardial infarction, is a serious condition in which part of the heart muscle dies. It occurs as the result of a blockage in the blood supply that provides the heart muscle with essential oxygen and nutrients.

In most cases, a heart attack is caused by the formation of a blood clot in one of the coronary arteries which encircle the heart. The clot characteristically develops in a section of the artery that is already narrowed by fatty deposits, a condition known as atherosclerosis. Less commonly, temporary spasm in the muscle wall of a coronary artery causes the obstruction.

Over 60,000 (officially recorded) deaths from heart attacks occur each year in the UK, making this by far the most common cause of death, with well over half this number being men. Roughly one man in 12 will die of a heart attack before he reaches retirement age. Risk factors for a heart attack are divided into those you can and those you cannot do something about.

Unavoidable risk factors include being male, getting older, a family history of heart attacks or abnormally high blood cholesterol, or suffering from diabetes or high blood pressure. Avoidable risk factors are smoking, drinking too much alcohol, not taking enough exercise, being overweight and eating a diet rich in saturated fat, cholesterol and sugary foods.

Symptoms of a heart attack may include pain across the centre of the chest – typically a severe crushing discomfort lasting for at least 20 minutes – pain spreading into the neck, jaw, shoulders or arms, sweating, nausea, vomiting, palpitations, dizziness and breathlessness.

Anyone suspected of having a heart attack should be seen by a doctor as soon as possible. Most heart attack deaths occur in the first few minutes and at least some could have been prevented if the appropriate first-aid measures had been carried out. It is therefore important to learn life-saving techniques, such as artificial ventilation and external cardiac compression, from a professional instructor, in case you have to help a heart attack victim whose breathing and heartbeat have stopped. A delay of even a few minutes while waiting for medical assistance is likely to prove fatal.

A new type of medication is now available which, injected into the circulation, can quickly dissolve the blood clots that cause most heart attacks. These 'clot-busting' drugs, such as streptokinase, can halt a heart attack and minimise heart muscle damage, as long as they are injected within a few hours of the onset of symptoms. Doctors also usually recommend daily low-dose aspirin therapy, which by thinning the blood can assist recovery and reduce the risk of later complications.

In addition, painrelieving drugs will be given, as well as drugs to treat any of the complications that may develop in more serious cases, such as heart failure or an irregular heartbeat. Surgical treatment of the blockage, following a heart attack, may include balloon angioplasty or coronary artery bypass grafting (see 'Angina', pages 187–8).

To assist recovery after a heart attack, ask your doctor for clear guidelines on returning to normal activities, including sex. As a general rule, sexual intercourse can be resumed once you can comfortably climb two flights of stairs. Doctors now encourage heart attack patients to follow a graded exercise programme, assuming there are no medical factors that make this too risky. Regular physical activity after a heart attack has been shown to reduce the chance of a recurrence.

Heartburn

Heartburn is an extremely common symptom. This painful burning sensation under your breastbone can vary from a niggling discomfort to a pain so intense it may be mistaken for a heart attack. Often heartburn sufferers also complain of belching and a bloated feeling because they subconsciously swallow air in an attempt to relieve their discomfort.

Some men develop heartburn as a reaction to a particular food: for example, rich, fatty or spicy meals are often to blame, as well as acidic fruits and vegetables, like grapefruit and tomatoes. Excessive chewing of gum may also bring on heartburn.

Recurrent episodes of heartburn may be caused by regurgitation of stomach acids into the oesophagus (gullet). A backflow of stomach acids can occur when the muscular valve which prevents this acid reflux is put under too much pressure as a result of, for example, overeating or being overweight. Carbonated drinks such as sparkling mineral water may bring on heartburn by raising pressure inside the stomach; coffee, smoking and alcohol may all provoke acid reflux by relaxing the valve.

Another cause for the valve not closing properly is a hiatus hernia, a common condition in which part of the stomach protrudes upwards into the chest cavity through a weakness in the diaphragm.

Typically, heartburn comes on within one hour of eating when stomach acid production peaks to aid digestion. Bending forwards, lying down and exercising too soon after a meal can also bring on an attack.

To help prevent heartburn:

- eat several small meals a day, and don't eat just before going to bed
- try to identify and avoid foods that bring on the pain
- cut down on alcohol, particularly neat spirits, and stop smoking
- don't bend over, lie down or exercise within one hour of eating
- try to lose any excess weight
- don't wear a tight belt or other restrictive clothing
- sleep with extra pillows, or elevate the bed head using 15-cm blocks
- take an antacid immediately after a meal.

See your doctor if you are suffering from persistent or recurrent heartburn and these measures have not worked. You may be prescribed a drug to reduce the amount of acid produced in the stomach, or a drug that tightens the muscular valve. In severe cases, surgery may be needed to strengthen the valve or repair a hiatus hernia.

Heart failure

This is a potentially serious condition in which the heart muscle is no longer able to pump efficiently. Although heart failure only rarely occurs in men under the age of 65, about 5 per cent of men in their 70s and 10 per cent of men over the age of 80 are affected.

Failure of the heart muscle pump is often the result of direct damage to the muscle fibres, following a heart attack or due to long-standing high blood pressure, for example. Other possible causes include a heart-valve defect, irregular heartbeat or excessive stimulation of the heart due to an overactive thyroid gland. Any long-standing lung disease which impedes the flow of blood, such as chronic bronchitis or emphysema, can also lead to heart failure by putting extra strain on the muscle wall of the right ventricle.

Initially, the heart may compensate for its decreased pumping ability through activation of the sympathetic nervous system (see pages 31–2), along with the release of the hormone renin in the kidneys, which in turn stimulates the production of a substance known as angiotensin II, which constricts the blood vessels. However, these changes are usually unable to maintain normal blood flow indefinitely and start to contribute themselves to a further deterioration in heart function.

Symptoms of heart failure typically include breathlessness, made worse by exertion or lying flat, muscle fatigue, swelling of the ankles and, sometimes, abdominal discomfort due to engorgement of the liver. In addition to carrying out a physical examination, the doctor may confirm the diagnosis by arranging a chest X-ray, electro-cardiogram (see Glossary) and an echocardiogram (ultrasound scan of the heart).

Drugs commonly used to treat heart failure include diuretics (which reduce fluid retention by increasing the volume of urine passed each day), an ACE inhibitor (which reduces the production of angiotensin II, improves blood flow and partially restores heart muscle function), digoxin (which stimulates the heart muscle to strengthen the power of its contractions) and a vasodilator (which eases the heart's workload by widening blood vessels around the body).

Finally, there are a number of self-help measures which may be recommended for someone who is suffering from heart failure, such as:

- raising the head of the bed to assist breathing
- gently exercising to improve heart and circulation function
- reducing salt consumption, which may otherwise encourage fluid retention
- elevating the feet when sitting to reduce ankle swelling
- losing excess weight to reduce strain on the heart.

Hernia

An abdominal hernia is the abnormal protrusion of an internal organ, usually part of the intestine, or fat, through a weakness in the abdominal muscle wall. This type of hernia is most common in older men, whose abdominal muscles tend to lose some of their strength and tone, partly due to them being less active and partly the result of putting on weight around the abdomen later in life.

If you notice a bulge in your abdominal wall, groin or scrotum see your doctor. The main risk from an abdominal hernia is obstruction of the intestine or its blood supply due to the protruding loop becoming compressed, which in turn can lead to potentially fatal complications.

Surgical repair is recommended in most cases to prevent complications occurring in the future. The operation is usually relatively easy for the surgeon to perform, taking about half an hour to complete and only keeping you in hospital for a few days at the most. Before returning to normal activities, particularly those which involve carrying or lifting, it is essential to follow a supervised programme of exercises to stretch and strengthen the abdominal muscles – otherwise, the risk of recurrence is much greater.

For those men who are not fit enough to have an operation, a surgical truss or corset may be provided to prevent the hernia from bulging through the muscle wall. For this to be effective, it must be possible to gently ease the hernia back inside the abdomen; the truss should be put on before getting out of bed and then worn all day.

If a hernia suddenly becomes painful, tender, swollen or inflamed, seek medical attention at once as these are signs that the intestine is under pressure.

High blood pressure

Everyone has blood pressure: this is the force that pushes blood through your arteries generated by the pumping action of the heart. The measurement of blood pressure comes as two figures: the higher reading is recorded at the moment the heart beats and the lower reading between beats when the heart muscle is relaxed.

Blood pressure varies throughout the day, increasing as a result of stress, exercise or pain and decreasing during periods of rest and relaxation. In a group of men, blood pressure measurements taken at rest will differ between individuals in the same way that their height and weight differ. The definition of high blood pressure is a reading above the accepted normal range, which according to the latest British Hypertension Society guidelines is 140/90.

Before a diagnosis of high blood pressure is made, usually a resting value of greater than 140/90 must have been recorded on at least three occasions. Healthy young men would normally have a blood pressure well below this threshold, with an average reading of 120/80. Older men are more likely to develop high blood pressure because their arteries have become less elastic and narrowed by deposits of fat (atherosclerosis).

High blood pressure almost always develops without any underlying medical cause, although in a few cases the blood pressure has been pushed up by a kidney, blood vessel or hormonal disorder. Certain medicines, such as anti-inflammatory drugs, can also increase your blood pressure. The medical term for high blood pressure is hypertension, but tension (stress) is only one possible contributory factor.

Most people with high blood pressure feel perfectly well and don't have any symptoms. The condition is usually only discovered during a routine test. Occasionally, high blood pressure causes headaches, dizziness, nausea or blurred vision, but these symptoms usually have some other explanation.

Because untreated high blood pressure can result in a number of serious complications, you should have your blood pressure routinely checked by your GP or practice nurse at least every five years and annually over the age of 55. These complications include thickening of the heart muscle and damage to arteries, particularly in the heart, brain, kidneys and eyes, thereby increasing the risk of heart failure, heart attack, stroke, kidney failure and loss of vision (due to haemorrhage in the retina at the back of the eye).

Not everyone with high blood pressure needs drug treatment. Measures to help correct high blood pressure include losing excess weight, taking regular exercise, eating a high-fibre, low-fat diet, cutting down on salt, restricting alcohol intake and stopping smoking. Relaxation and meditation can also help. Avoid activities that cause a prolonged build-up of tension in the muscles, such as heavy lifting and powerful gripping, as these can lead to a big increase in blood pressure. If blood pressure remains high despite these measures, there are several different types of antihypertensive drug your doctor can choose from, including diuretics, beta blockers, ACE inhibitors and calcium channel blockers.

Indigestion

The term indigestion is used to describe a number of different types of symptom related to the digestive system and brought on by eating or drinking, for example nausea, heartburn (see pages 235–6), wind, feeling bloated, or discomfort in the upper abdomen. Almost everyone suffers from the occasional attack of indigestion.

In many cases, indigestion is simply the result of eating too much, eating too fast, eating hot, spicy or fatty food, drinking too much alcohol or being under stress. Taking an antacid or an H_2 antagonist, such as Pepcid, Zantac or Tagamet, available from the pharmacy, will usually relieve symptoms rapidly.

However, if you suffer from recurrent attacks of indigestion, you should see a doctor as you might have some underlying disorder of the digestive tract, such as gastritis (inflammation of the stomach), a peptic ulcer (see pages 258–9), irritable bowel syndrome (see pages 241–2) or gallstones (see pages 226–7).

If abdominal pain persists for more than six hours or you develop other symptoms, such as persistent vomiting or passing dark or black faeces, you should seek immediate medical attention.

Ingrown toenail

An ingrown toenail is a painful condition, usually affecting one or both of the big toes, in which the edge of the nail or a nail splinter is pressing down into the skin to cause inflammation and sometimes infection. This condition, which is most common in young men between the ages of 16 and 25, is usually the result of cutting the nail incorrectly or wearing tight fitting shoes.

You should cut your toenails straight across to avoid damaging the corners and exposing vulnerable skin. If your shoes are too narrow they can put pressure on the nail and, by encouraging your feet to sweat more, will soften the adjacent skin, making it easier for it to be pierced by a nail splinter or the edge of the nail.

If the edge of one of your toenails becomes painful, red and swollen bathe your feet twice daily in warm, salty water and, after drying, cover the nail with dry gauze dressing.

If the symptoms do not settle down, you may need to take a course of antibiotics. You should also make an appointment to see a chiropodist as you may need minor surgery, either to remove a splinter of nail or to remove a narrow section of the nail edge and destroy the nail bed underneath it, allowing the nail to grow back normally.

Insomnia

People vary a great deal in the amount of sleep they need to wake up feeling rested and refreshed and, as you get older, you are likely to require less sleep. Some individuals seem to be able to manage on only four hours a night, while others complain that even with ten they still feel washed out.

Insomnia is not just being unable to sleep for as long as you want. Sleep may be very fitful causing you to wake feeling out of sorts and tired; you may take a long time to fall asleep, or may wake up in the early hours of the morning and be unable to fall asleep again. If you suffer from insomnia, try some of the following measures to alleviate the problem:

- take some exercise during the day, preferably in the fresh air, so that you feel tired at bedtime
- have a light meal early in the evening. If you eat a large meal within a couple of hours of going to bed, an active digestive system is likely to keep you awake

- don't drink a late cup of tea or coffee that contains the stimulant caffeine; have a decaffeinated or warm milky drink instead
- alcohol can interfere with sleep, so drink it only in moderation
- if you are working late, take at least an hour off to unwind before you go to bed
- have a warm bath to help you relax
- make sure the bedroom isn't too hot or too cold and if there is a background noise that you can't sleep through, such as traffic or your partner snoring, try using earplugs
- sleep on a firm but comfortable mattress
- get up at the same time each morning regardless of how well you slept
- if you are elderly, try having a short nap during the day – paradoxically, this may improve your night's sleep
- don't worry if you can't get to sleep: just resting in bed will be doing you some good
- at bedtime read for pleasure, not work or study.

See your doctor if your insomnia persists despite these measures. If you are under a lot of stress, or feeling anxious about something in your life, your doctor may recommend some form of muscle relaxation or breathing exercise to help you get off to sleep. Nowadays, you will normally be prescribed a sedative only as a last resort. A drug-induced sleep is not as restful and it is easy to become dependent on this type of drug, with unpleasant withdrawal symptoms if you stop it suddenly.

It may be that you need to take sleeping tablets for a few days to help you get back into your normal sleeping pattern if you are going through a particularly bad time. However, to avoid becoming dependent, it is best not to use sleeping tablets every night for longer than a week. Also, they tend to become less effective with regular use.

Irritable bowel syndrome

Irritable bowel syndrome is a disorder of the bowel muscle function. Although there is no specific physical abnormality, such as inflammation or an ulcer or tumour, this condition can produce distressing symptoms. Sufferers from an irritable bowel may complain of a wide variety of symptoms, ranging from colicky abdominal cramps, usually low down on the left side, excess gas, abdominal swelling and a bloated feeling and alternating bouts of diarrhoea and constipation, to nausea, vomiting, loss of appetite and extreme lethargy.

The recurrent abdominal pains are typically worse soon after eating a meal and ease off after passing wind or faeces.

As many as one in three of the population in the UK will suffer occasional symptoms of an irritable bowel (symptoms usually begin to cause problems between the ages of 15 and 40 years). One in ten people develops symptoms bad enough to consult a doctor.

Stress can certainly be one aggravating factor, but it is not the only cause. In fact, many men with irritable bowel syndrome have no problems with stress, anxiety or depression. When stress is playing a part, counselling and relaxation techniques can do more to relieve symptoms than any drug treatment.

Another important factor is diet. Some sufferers react badly to certain foods, such as wheat, dairy products and citrus fruits; simply identifying and avoiding these foods may be enough to ease the symptoms. About one-third of people with an irritable bowel benefit from slowly increasing their intake of high-fibre foods, such as fresh fruit and vegetables, wholegrain bread and cereals, rice and pulses. However, many others are made worse by this type of diet and should try a low-fibre diet.

It is also advisable to cut down on tea and coffee, but make sure you drink at least eight glasses of non-carbonated water each day, as fluids help maintain good bowel function. Take a laxative only if your doctor recommends one; in fact, an irritant laxative, such as senna, can make the pains worse.

See your doctor if you have persistent or recurrent symptoms; do not just assume you have this condition: a check-up is necessary to rule out more serious bowel disorders. You may be prescribed peppermint oil capsules or an antispasmodic drug to relax painful bowel muscle spasm, or a bulking laxative to soften and increase the volume of your stools.

Jaundice

Jaundice is the yellowing of the skin and the whites of the eyes caused by a build up of the yellow-brown-coloured bile pigment in the blood. The urine may also appear abnormally dark as this pigment is passed out of the body through the kidneys.

Bile pigment is produced from haemoglobin (the oxygen-carrying substance inside red blood cells), when old red blood cells are broken down, mainly by the spleen. Red blood cells normally last only about 120 days and are continually being replaced by new red blood cells made inside the bone marrow (see page 45). This bile pigment is absorbed from the blood into the liver, where it is itself broken down and passed though the bile ducts into the small bowel to assist in the digestion of fatty foods. Jaundice occurs when this process is upset in one of the following ways:

- excessive destruction of red blood cells, caused by certain bugs, such as malaria, and certain drugs
- liver disease, which interferes with the transfer of bile pigment to the bile ducts, e.g. hepatitis (see pages 124–5)
- blockage of the bile ducts e.g. by gallstones (see pages 226–7).

Anyone developing jaundice will need urgent medical attention so that the underlying cause can be diagnosed and treated accordingly.

Klinefelter's syndrome

Klinefelter's syndrome is a rare chromosome abnormality in which a male is born with one or more extra X chromosomes in his cells, resulting in a chromosome pattern of XXY, or more rarely XXXY or XXXXY, rather than the normal XY. This syndrome affects about one in every 750 male infants born in the UK. The risk of having a baby affected by Kleinfelter's syndrome increases with the age of the mother.

The features of Kleinfelter's syndrome vary in severity and may become apparent only at puberty, when breast enlargement (gynaecomastia) may develop and the testes remain small and hard. Affected males tend to be tall and thin, with a body shape that looks more female than male. The majority will be infertile due to a complete absence of sperm production. However, occasionally, when a mosaic pattern of chromosomes is present, with some of the cells showing the normal XY pattern, the man may be fertile.

The incidence of mental retardation is higher in men with Kleifelter's syndrome than in the general population. Other associated disorders include autism and diabetes mellitus. Affected men also have a greater risk of developing testicular and breast cancer.

Diagnosis is confirmed by a chromosome analysis using white blood cells taken from a blood sample. Testosterone replacement therapy in the form of an implant or skin patch may be prescribed to induce the development of secondary sexual characteristics, such as growth of facial and pubic hair, to increase sex drive and to help prevent future osteoporosis (see pages 251–3).

Laryngitis

Laryngitis is a condition in which the larynx (voice box) becomes inflamed. Symptoms may include a dry and irritating cough, pain or discomfort in the throat, which is typically made worse by swallowing, and hoarseness sometimes progressing to a complete loss of voice.

Acute laryngitis comes on suddenly and lasts only a few days. The most common cause is a viral infection, such as a cold, in which case the individual will usually have a fever and feel unwell. Occasionally, acute laryngitis develops as a result of an allergic reaction to pollen or to some other substance.

Chronic laryngitis develops more slowly and can last for several weeks or months. The most common cause is overusing the voice, for example while coaching a sports team. Other possible reasons include trauma during a bout of violent coughing or irritation from prolonged exposure to cigarette smoke.

Anyone who develops the symptoms of laryngitis should rest their voice as much as possible and avoid smoking. Putting a humidifier or boiling a kettle in a room to fill it with steam can help ease the associated discomfort and cough. Paracetamol or aspirin (not in children under 12) should be taken to relieve any pain or fever.

If the symptoms are due to infection and persist for longer than a few days or if you start to cough up sputum, then you may need a course of antibiotics. If hoarseness persists for several weeks, then you may be referred to an ear, nose and throat specialist for examination of your vocal cords to check for nodules or tumours.

Meningitis

Meningitis is a serious, potentially fatal condition in which the membranes that form the outer lining over the brain and spinal cord (meninges) become inflamed, usually as a result of a viral or bacterial infection. The bugs that cause meningitis usually reach the meninges via the bloodstream, having been carried there from another part of the body. However, occasionally the bugs come through the skull from a sinus or ear infection or from the air following a skull fracture.

Viral meningitis, which tends to occur in epidemics during the winter and may be mistaken for an attack of 'flu, usually clears up within two weeks and does not leave any after-effects. Bacterial meningitis is potentially a lot more serious, particularly the form known as meningococcal meningitis, which carries a risk of permanent brain damage and even death.

Symptoms of meningitis may include headache, neck stiffness, dislike of bright light, vomiting, fever and sometimes drowsiness and confusion. In meningococcal meningitis, the symptoms come on rapidly and are often accompanied by a rash consisting of tiny reddish-purple spots or bruises, and drowsiness may progress to loss of consciousness.

Anyone who develops symptoms characteristic of meningitis should be seen by a doctor immediately. Diagnosis is confirmed by lumbar puncture, in which a small amount of spinal fluid is removed through a needle inserted into the lower back. When meningitis is due to a viral infection, treatment is simply rest and painkillers until the symptoms clear up. Bacterial meningitis requires immediate treatment with high doses of antibiotics to reduce the risk of brain damage and death.

Vaccination to protect against meningitis is effective only with specific types of bug and, because it is effective only for a short time, it is only worth being immunised during an epidemic. Anyone who has been in recent contact with an individual with bacterial meningitis can be protected by receiving a course of antibiotics.

Migraine

A typical migraine attack causes a throbbing headache, usually on one side of the head, with nausea and vomiting. Visual disturbances, such as seeing flashing lights or zigzag shapes, or partial loss of vision, may also occur, sometimes just before the onset of headache. Occasionally, an attack may cause numbness and tingling in the limbs and increased sensitivity to light and noise.

For many sufferers, a migraine attack can mean several hours of excruciating pain that makes it impossible to work or even think straight, followed by a day or more of feeling totally exhausted.

Ordinary painrelievers often don't seem to help much, and the only solution is to retreat to a darkened room and try to sleep until the symptoms ease off.

Although the exact cause of migraine remains unknown, the throbbing headache is thought to be due to a temporary widening of blood vessels in the brain and scalp. Some people are able to identify and then avoid specific trigger factors that provoke an attack, such as missing a meal, not drinking enough water, sleeping in longer than usual, or eating a specific type of food over the previous two days.

Eating regularly, avoiding lying in (at the weekend or on holiday), and cutting out cheese, chocolate, oranges, peanut butter and certain alcoholic drinks such as red wine or spirits may help reduce the frequency of attacks. Unfortunately, however, the majority of migraine sufferers are unable to find such an easy solution.

If ordinary painrelievers, such as aspirin or paracetamol, on their own or combined with codeine, fail to improve your headache, an anti-inflammatory drug such as ibuprofen, which you can buy from the pharmacist, may help. Whatever brand of painreliever you use, it is important to take it as soon as you feel an attack coming on to get the best effect. Soluble or effervescent preparations are preferable because they work quicker.

See your doctor if you are suffering from frequent disabling attacks of migraine. You may be prescribed a preventive drug, such as a betablocker or sanomigran, which can stop migraine coming on but won't help an acute attack. However, although these drugs are often effective, they commonly cause side-effects – betablockers are associated with lethargy and sanomigran with weight gain. A relatively new class of prescription drugs, known as selective $5HT_1$ agonists, are able to relieve migraine symptoms rapidly in most people. They work primarily by narrowing the blood vessels in the brain and scalp that become abnormally dilated during a migraine attack. Examples of these new drugs include zolmitriptan, naratriptan and sumatriptan, the latter available as a self-administered injection and nasal spray, as well as being taken by mouth. However, because they also narrow the blood vessels inside the heart muscle, selective $5HT_1$ agonists should not be taken by people with heart disease, such as angina.

Regular use of feverfew, a herbal preparation, has been shown to reduce the frequency of migraine attacks and decrease the severity of nausea and vomiting during an attack. Although you can grow your own feverfew plants, or buy feverfew tablets from a pharmacy or health store, it is best to consult a qualified herbal practitioner for advice on the correct dose for you.

A few people seem to be helped by acupuncture or hypnotherapy and, because stress can trigger migraine, it is worth trying relaxation exercises (see Chapter 3), which may help control attacks by reducing tension.

Multiple sclerosis

Multiple sclerosis (MS) is a disease of the nervous system in which the outer lining (myelin) that covers some of the nerve fibres in the brain and spinal cord becomes damaged and scarred. As a result of this damage, the transfer of messages through the brain and nervous system is disrupted.

Although the exact cause of MS remains unknown, this condition is thought to be an auto-immune disease in which the body's immune system starts to attack its own tissues, in this case myelin. The trigger for this attack may be a previous viral infection. The cause may also be genetic as close relatives of someone with MS are eight times more likely to develop the disease themselves.

The incidence of MS in the UK is roughly one in every 1,000 people, usually starting in early adult life. Symptoms of MS may include double vision, dizziness and loss of balance, numbness, tingling, clumsiness, weakness, tremor and incontinence. Each of these symptoms may occur on its own or in combination with others. Typically an attack lasts a few weeks or months and then the symptoms go away for a long period.

In some cases MS strikes only once and never returns. However, for the majority of sufferers, the occurrence of a second episode means that intermittent attacks will then return for the rest of their life. Months or even years may pass between attacks, but usually the intervals become progressively shorter. In addition, it is likely that they will be left with some residual disability in between times of increasing severity.

While the course of MS is highly varied and unpredictable, certain factors seem to bring on an attack, such as injury, infection or emotional stress. Some people are able to return to work and lead normal lives between attacks, while others may become confined to a wheelchair and need nursing care.

The diagnosis of MS is made by excluding other nervous system diseases using X-rays and other imaging procedures such as MRI or CT scans, along with electrical tests to measure the speed of impulses along different nerve pathways.

Treatment may include high doses of corticosteroids during an attack, which can reduce the severity of symptoms, and physiotherapy to help improve muscle strength, balance and mobility. Recently, a new class of drugs – the interferons beta-1a and beta-1b – has been developed, which appears to reduce the frequency and severity of relapses in some people by suppressing the damaging effect of the immune system on myelin. For further information, contact the Multiple Sclerosis Society.*

Mumps

Once a common childhood disease, mumps now occurs only rarely since the introduction of routine immunisation of young children against this viral infection. Symptoms of mumps include painful swelling of the salivary glands on one or both sides of the upper neck and under the jaw, difficulty chewing and swallowing, along with fever and loss of appetite.

Before immunisation, mumps used to spread quickly through schools and other communities. The incubation period between exposure to the mumps virus and the onset of the symptoms is two to three weeks. An infected person can pass on the mumps virus to others in saliva droplets through coughing and sneezing for about one week before and for up to two weeks after his symptoms appear.

A mumps vaccine was introduced for several reasons. Although mumps causes only a mild illness that lasts for up to 10 days in most children, the infection may very rarely spread to the brain and spinal cord, causing encephalitis and/or meningitis (see pages 244–5), which occasionally leads to permanent deafness. Pancreatitis (inflammation of the pancreas), causing severe abdominal pain and vomiting, may also develop as a complication of mumps, most commonly in adolescents and adults.

Also, in young men post puberty, mumps may cause an attack of orchitis, in which one or rarely both testicles becomes extremely painful, tender and swollen for several days. Mumps orchitis is treated with painkillers and sometimes a short course of corticosteroids to reduce the inflammation. Although the affected testicle may shrink a little afterwards, this will not usually cause infertility by interfering with sperm production unless both testicles are affected.

At one time doctors gave an immunoglobulin shot to adult men if they started to develop mumps symptoms, but this is no longer done because there is no evidence that it reduces the risk of complications such as orchitis.

Myalgic encephalomyelitis (ME)

This mysterious disease, which usually strikes people in their late 20s or early 30s, is characterised by severe physical and mental exhaustion. Symptoms may include extreme muscle fatigue, muscle pains like hundreds of pinpricks, aching joints, headaches, disturbed sleep, loss of memory, difficulty concentrating, dizziness and blurred vision.

ME is also referred to as chronic fatigue syndrome, but it is more than just ordinary tiredness. During this illness, even the simplest activities, such as walking from room to room, require a tremendous effort. A typical description likens ME to having a severe bout of 'flu which seems to go on for ever. Symptoms can persist for several years, with intermittent periods of recovery interspersed with episodes of sudden relapse. However, most ME sufferers will make a full recovery eventually.

The exact cause is unknown, but experts believe that symptoms are brought on by an abnormal response to a viral infection, which in turn disrupts the function of the muscles and nerves. Many ME sufferers pinpoint the onset of their condition as a specific infection, usually of the throat or chest.

There is no conventional drug treatment for ME. Antidepressants were often prescribed in the past, but depression is thought to be a consequence rather than a cause of ME. Recovery from ME can be assisted and the chances of a relapse reduced by the following measures:

- drinking little or no alcohol
- cutting down on highly refined carbohydrate (sugary) foods
- avoiding extremes of temperature
- undergoing immunisation or a general anaesthetic only if essential
- taking an adequate period of complete rest
- gradually returning to normal activities over several months
- exercising gently and regularly, but never pushing yourself too hard.

Some ME sufferers are helped by alternative therapies such as homoeopathy, herbal medicine and aromatherapy. Recently, thermoregulatory hydrotherapy (TRHT), a technique in which the patient undergoes gradual immersion in cold water at a temperature of 16°C, has been shown to make a significant difference to symptoms after several weeks of daily exposure.

Obesity

The standard method used to define the terms overweight and obesity is to take the individual's body weight, measured in kilograms, and divide it by the square of his height in metres ($W \div H^2$). This formula produces a figure known as the body mass index (BMI – see pages 70–1).

A man with a BMI between 25 and 30 is defined as being overweight, although occasionally this slightly higher than normal figure may be due to muscle bulk rather than fat. A BMI above 30 is defined as obesity.

In the UK, about 10 per cent of men over the age of 40 are obese. The cause in most cases is a combination of overeating and not taking enough exercise to burn off excess calories. Your weight will remain stable only if your energy intake in the form of calories from food and drink is in balance with the energy expended to keep your body organs ticking over at rest, as well as fuelling your muscles when you exercise. Any excess supply of energy is converted into fat stores, which in men are mainly deposited around the abdomen as a paunch.

In addition to unhealthy eating and exercise habits, obesity also tends to run in families. If both your parents are or were obese, you stand a much greater chance of becoming obese yourself. However, this may not just be a genetic phenomenon, as an unhealthy lifestyle can also be passed on from one generation to the next.

A few men – the so-called 'underburners' – need fewer calories to satisfy their daily energy needs, and therefore have to be extra careful to keep their weight under control.

Older men are more vulnerable to becoming overweight or obese because their energy requirement gradually decreases. The loss of muscle tissue that occurs as a normal part of ageing means the body needs less energy for muscle cell metabolism at rest. Also, older men tend to take less physical exercise and therefore burn up fewer calories overall. Because it is difficult to change eating habits, the necessary gradual reduction in daily calorie intake to keep the balance between energy supply and demand is not made. As a result, fat will slowly build up and weight will steadily increase with advancing years.

Being overweight can be a serious hazard to your health. Not only will you tend to become tired and breathless more easily, but you will also be more vulnerable to a wide variety of medical disorders, including back pain, osteoarthritis, varicose veins, gallstones and even certain types of cancer, such as cancer of the colon, rectum and prostate. Obesity also increases the risk of high blood pressure, high blood cholesterol and diabetes, all of which are associated with a greater chance of suffering from a heart attack or stroke.

To prevent or control obesity, you need to pay attention to your diet and take regular exercise. Suitable diet and exercise programmes for men who are overweight are described in detail in Chapter 2.

Osteoarthritis

Osteoarthritis, the most common form of arthritis, is the result of wear and tear of the cartilage surfaces inside a joint causing pain, stiffness and swelling. This wearing out of the joint tends to occur gradually with advancing years. Most men in their 60s have osteoarthritis in at least some of their joints.

The joints most commonly affected are those that have taken the most punishment over the years – the hips, the knees and the joints at the base of the neck and lower back. Factors which increase the risk of osteoarthritis include being overweight, overuse of a joint playing a particular sport, or a serious or recurrent injury to a joint when younger.

There is no cure for osteoarthritis, but symptoms can usually be controlled with painrelievers, or anti-inflammatory drugs taken by mouth or applied to the affected joints as a gel. A doctor or physiotherapist may be able to recommend exercises to strengthen the muscles around an arthritic joint, which should also help to protect the joint against further damage.

In severe cases, where the arthritic joint has become very painful or stiff, sufferers may be referred to hospital for a joint-replacement operation.

Osteoporosis

Osteoporosis is a bone disorder in which the density of the bones decreases, causing them to become more brittle and vulnerable to fracture. The first sign is often a fracture from a fall that would not normally be severe enough to break a bone. Typical sites for these fractures are the wrist and top of the thighbone (femur). In addition, weakening of the vertebral bones due to osteoporosis may cause them to crumble, resulting in loss of height, deformity of the spine and occasionally pain from pressure on a spinal nerve.

Diagnosis may be confirmed from bone X-rays, as well as scanning techniques, which measure bone density. Blood tests and a bone biopsy may be carried out to exclude other bone disorders.

Some risk factors for osteoporosis are beyond control, such as your sex, race and genes. For example, men are less at risk of osteoporosis than women but they can still develop this condition, particularly white men with a family history of osteoporosis. In fact, one fifth of all osteoporosis sufferers are men, and one in six men will suffer an osteoporosis-related fracture before the age of 90.

Although osteoporosis occurs as a natural part of ageing, a number of preventive measures can be taken to reduce the severity of the condition. These measures are based on ensuring that good quality, strong and dense bone forms while the bones are still actively growing and maturing in early adulthood, and then minimising the influence ageing has on causing a progressive loss of protein from the bone structure. These preventive measures include:

- **taking exercise** – regular physical activity maximises the density of your bones while they are still growing and maturing and then minimises bone loss later in life
- **stopping smoking and heavy drinking** – as both these habits increase the risk of developing osteoporosis
- **adequate calcium intake** – this is essential to grow and maintain strong healthy bones. If your diet is deficient in calcium, hormonal changes will occur automatically within your body to withdraw calcium from your bones to maintain levels of this chemical in the bloodstream. Foods rich in calcium include milk and milk products, green leafy vegetables, citrus fruits, sardines and shellfish. To maintain a satisfactory intake of calcium without consuming excessive amounts of saturated fat, drink semi-skimmed milk and stick to low fat yoghurts and cheeses. Anyone with a family history of kidney stones, or who has suffered from kidney stones in the past, should have blood tests to ensure that he does not already have an

abnormally high level of calcium in his bloodstream before deliberately increasing his intake of this mineral

- **vitamin D** – because vitamin D helps facilitate the absorption of calcium from digested food, it is also important to maintain an adequate intake of this nutrient in your diet. Most men will get all the vitamin D they need from foods such as low fat spreads and oily fish. However, your doctor may advise taking a vitamin D supplement in addition to extra calcium.

For men who have started to develop osteoporosis, treatment with injections of a synthetic form of the thyroid hormone calcitonin can prevent further bone loss by blocking the action of parathyroid hormone, which speeds up the rate of calcium loss from the bones. Alternatively, one of a new class of drugs – the biphosphonates – which inhibits the dissolving of calcium crystals, as well as blocking the activity of cells responsible for bone reabsorption, may be prescribed. For further information, contact the National Osteoporosis Society.*

Panic attacks

Panic attacks are brief episodes of intense anxiety, characterised by a strong feeling that something terrible or frightening is about to happen, or a fear of going crazy. As many as two per cent of men suffer from recurrent panic attacks, which occur unpredictably and for no apparent reason.

Symptoms typically come on suddenly and may include shaking, sweating, palpitations, nausea and a sensation of choking, tightness across the chest, dizziness or light-headedness. During an attack, the person may feel that the outside world is no longer real or that he has become detached from reality, like being in a dream. Hyperventilation (fast, shallow breathing) often accompanies a panic attack and worsens the symptoms, causing numbness and tingling around the mouth and in the hands and feet.

The symptoms of a panic attack are the result of the body's natural response to stress, anxiety or fear. They are part of the primitive 'fight or flight' mechanism in which survival depends on the efficient activation of the heart, lungs, muscles and circulation, enabling an individual to escape from or defend himself against any threat to his life. A panic attack is simply the result of over-activation of this response, causing the symptoms to become intense and uncontrolled.

Some people are simply prone to above average levels of anxiety. However, in others, the onset of panic attacks can be traced back to a particularly stressful experience, even though the symptoms now appear unrelated to this original trauma. Often, simply the fear of a panic attack coming on is enough to start the symptoms off. In contrast to a phobia, this panic reaction is not related directly to any specific object or situation.

Although panic attacks may be extremely unpleasant and frightening, they are not dangerous and do not cause any long-term physical harm. Even if nothing is done to stop an attack, the symptoms will soon pass. For many sufferers, this explanation and reassurance is often enough to reduce significantly the frequency and severity of their panic attacks.

Measures that can help you include regular relaxation exercises, particularly a routine that encourages controlled deep breathing (see pages 112–13) to suppress the tendency to hyperventilate during an attack. If you do start to hyperventilate, you should breathe slowly in and out of a small paper bag held over your mouth and nose. This technique reduces the amount of carbon dioxide being blown off from the lungs and, as a result, prevents the upset in blood chemistry that otherwise makes the symptoms a lot worse.

If, despite the above actions, your panic attacks remain uncontrolled, behaviour therapy or psychotherapy may be recommended. Also, you may benefit from taking a type of antidepressant, which raises the level of the brain chemical serotonin. Tranquillisers are only rarely prescribed nowadays to treat or prevent a panic attack because they do not solve the underlying problem and they carry a risk of addiction if they are taken regularly for more than a week.

Parkinson's disease

Parkinson's disease is a disorder of the nervous system resulting from degeneration of part of the brain known as the basal ganglia, which controls movement and muscle tension. About one in 100 men over the age of 65 years, and one in 50 over the age of 80, develop this condition, although it can also occasionally affect younger men. Parkinsonism is the term used to describe any condition that mimics Parkinson's disease but which has a specific cause, such as a drug reaction or brain damage in a boxer from repeated blows to the head (punch-drunk syndrome).

Symptoms of Parkinson's disease may include shaking of one or both hands, stiff muscles, slow reactions and a fixed facial expression with staring, unblinking eyes. Typically, one side of the body is affected first and the symptoms become progressively more severe over many years. The shaking tends to be worse at rest and improves during movement.

Parkinson's disease can also have an effect on walking. The person will typically find it difficult to get started, walk with a marked stoop, and the steps he takes will be short and fast to avoid falling forwards. Although his speech may become slow and hesitant, intellectual function does not usually deteriorate until a late stage in the disease.

Although, as yet, Parkinson's disease cannot be cured, much can be done to minimise the disability it causes. In addition to physiotherapy, which helps to improve mobility, posture and independence, a variety of drug treatments are now often prescribed in combination. Because the benefits of these drugs may wear off with continuous use, regular review of medication is necessary, and the patient may be given different products.

The aim of drug treatment is to correct disturbances in the balance between two of the brain chemicals, dopamine and acetylcholine. Drugs that mimic or potentiate the action of dopamine help compensate for the reduced level of this chemical which exists as a result of the brain degeneration. Drugs that block the action of acetylcholine are effective at reducing specific symptoms, such as the tremor and stiffness, but do not help improve mobility.

A few people with Parkinson's disease may be referred for surgery, particularly if they are young and otherwise in good health. Transplantation of dopamine-secreting tissues, which have been taken either from the patient's own adrenal glands or from aborted foetuses, into the brain have significantly improved symptoms and reduced disability in some people. For further information, contact The Parkinson's Disease Society.★

Penis disorders

A wide variety of disorders can affect the penis. Penile warts, sexually transmitted diseases and the causes and treatment of erectile dysfunction are discussed in detail in Chapter 4. Other penis disorders include:

Balanitis The glans (head) of the penis and foreskin (if present) become inflamed, resulting in a red, moist appearance with itching or discomfort. It is usually caused by infection, either with bacteria or a fungus such as thrush, and treatment is likely to be the appropriate antibiotic or antifungal drug prescribed by your doctor.

Poor hygiene may play a part in causing the infection, but thrush is invariably picked up during sexual intercourse with an infected partner, who should therefore be treated as well.

Having an abnormally tight foreskin (phimosis), which is difficult or impossible to pull back, increases the risk of balanitis by preventing the man from washing under his foreskin properly. Most young boys have a tight foreskin, but this should not be forced back otherwise there is a risk that it will become damaged or stuck. Normally the foreskin becomes more mobile as the boy grows older, but if a phimosis persists and is causing either recurrent balanitis or pain during intercourse or masturbation, circumcision (see opposite) is usually recommended.

Occasionally, balanitis is due to irritation from residual laundry detergent on underpants, or an allergic reaction to a spermicide or condom.

Priapism This is a condition whereby erection becomes abnormally prolonged and sometimes painful in the absence of sexual arousal. It occurs when blood is unable to drain back out of the penis, for example due to nerve damage, a blood clotting disease or blocked circulation due to infection. Nowadays, the most common cause is a side-effect from the various drug treatments of erectile dysfunction (see pages 153–5).

Emergency treatment of priapism is essential to avoid permanent damage. This may be by injection of local anaesthetic into the spine, or by withdrawal of blood from the penis using a sterile needle and syringe.

Peyronie's disease Thickening of part of the fibrous sheath inside the penis causes it to bend at an alarming angle each time it becomes erect, making intercourse painful or impossible. This condition usually affects only men over the age of 40.

Although the exact cause of Peyronie's disease is unknown, it may be provoked by minor trauma to the penis during vigorous sexual activity. When the penis becomes flaccid, the thickened area may be felt as a firm nodule.

A few men require surgery to straighten the penis, which involves the insertion of special stitches on the opposite side to the bend.

Penile cancer   This extremely rare form of malignant tumour is more common in uncircumcised men and is associated with poor personal hygiene and smoking. The tumour usually first appears as a painless wart or a painful ulcer on the tip of the penis.

If diagnosed early, circumcision followed by radiotherapy may be successful without the need for further surgery. Therefore, always have an immediate check-up with your doctor if you develop any wart or ulcer on your penis that persists for over two weeks.

CIRCUMCISION

Surgical removal of the foreskin – circumcision – is a procedure in which the inner and outer layers of this flap of skin are cut away and the raw edges stitched together. This operation has been carried out for many centuries as a religious ritual on all male infants born into Jewish or Moslem families. Whereas in the past it would normally have been the rabbi or imam who performed the circumcision, it is now usually done by a surgeon, which should reduce the risk of complications, such as excessive bleeding or infection.

Non-religious circumcision began in the Victorian era, as a means of deliberately desensitising the penis to discourage masturbation. However, not only does circumcision not prevent masturbation, it also does not make any difference to hygiene.

Nowadays, it is much less fashionable to circumcise boys purely for hygienic reasons because there is no reason why an uncircumcised man should not keep himself clean by pulling back his foreskin to wash away any build-up of secretions (smegma) each day.

However, of the 30,000 circumcisions still being performed each year in the UK, at least some could be avoided. For example, ballooning of the foreskin during urination is normal in children as the foreskin starts to loosen up – this does not, on its own, require surgery.

Genuine medical reasons for circumcision in adult men include an abnormally tight foreskin (phimosis), which is causing pain when the penis is erect or during intercourse, or recurrent infection under the foreskin – a condition known as balanitis (see page 256).

In children and adults, circumcision is usually performed under a general anaesthetic. For the first 48 hours after the operation, intermittent application of an ice-pack may be recommended to reduce swelling and bruising. After that, a warm bath with a handful of table salt added to the water will help keep the wound clean. It may not be possible to wear underpants for a few days while the wound remains uncomfortable.

If you are an adult man advised to have a circumcision, or a parent considering having your son circumcised, you can get support and further information by contacting NORM UK.*

Peptic ulcer

The two main types of peptic ulcer are ulceration of the duodenum (duodenal ulcer or DU), which will develop in about one in ten people at some time in their lives, and a gastric (stomach) ulcer which occurs in about one in 30. Men are more likely to develop a duodenal ulcer than women, but the chances of a man or woman suffering from a gastric ulcer are about equal.

Both these forms of peptic ulcer usually first appear in middle age, but the peak age of onset for a DU is on average ten years earlier.

Typical symptoms of a peptic ulcer include a burning or gnawing pain in the abdomen, which will sometimes wake the sufferer at night. While the pain from a DU is characteristically relieved by eating, only to reappear a few hours later, the pain due to a gastric ulcer is made worse by food and drink. Other symptoms that may occur with both types of ulcer are loss of appetite, nausea, vomiting, belching, feeling bloated and loss of weight.

Many ulcer sufferers only become aware of their condition if they develop a complication, such as severe abdominal pain due to the ulcer perforating, or vomiting of blood material which looks like coffee grounds if the ulcer bleeds.

The ulcer may be diagnosed by gastroscopy, whereby a viewing instrument is passed through the mouth, down the oesophagus and into the stomach and duodenum. A barium X-ray examination, for which the patient drinks a solution of barium that shows up white on subsequent X-ray pictures, can also reveal both gastric and duodenal ulcers.

Thanks to advances in medical therapy, surgery for a peptic ulcer is usually reserved nowadays for those cases in which a complication has developed. In addition to antacids, which can relieve ulcer pain by decreasing stomach acidity, a range of powerful ulcer-healing drugs is now available.

A common problem, however, has been the large number of people who relapse within a year of their peptic ulcer being healed. One way to overcome this is to take a low dose of an ulcer-healing drug indefinitely.

A new approach to treatment, recently introduced, works on the basis that H. pylori, a particular type of bacterium found in the upper part of the digestive system, is responsible for the formation of almost all duodenal ulcers. If these bacteria are detected in a blood or breath test, they can be eradicated by taking a combination of two antibiotics and bismuth – a drug which also promotes ulcer healing – to achieve a long-term cure.

To reduce your chance of developing a peptic ulcer, or suffering a recurrence once an ulcer has healed:

- stop smoking and cut down on alcohol, coffee and tea
- eat small meals at regular intervals and avoid a large meal within two hours of going to bed
- choose a painreliever that contains paracetamol, with or without codeine, rather than aspirin or any other type of anti-inflammatory drug.

Piles (haemorrhoids)

Piles are swollen blood vessels in the lower part of the rectum and anal canal, similar to the varicose veins that many people develop in their legs (see pages 284–6). As many as 40 per cent of men will suffer from piles at some time in their lives, although many of them will never go for treatment because they are too embarrassed or shy.

The most common cause of piles is thought to be straining while passing stools. The risk is increased if the person is constipated, with hard bowel movements that take more time and effort to pass. Although piles usually first appear in middle age, in some people they may appear earlier because of an inherited weakness in the blood vessel walls. Ignore the old wives' tales which say that piles can be brought on by sitting on a hot radiator or on a cold or damp surface or by doing a job that involves sitting down all day. Symptoms include:

- bleeding during a bowel movement, which causes spots of blood to appear on the toilet bowl and toilet paper
- irritation around the anus
- slight mucous discharge.

Any bleeding from the anus should be checked out by a doctor. Although it is not usually due to any serious bowel disorder, it could be an early warning sign of bowel cancer, particularly if the blood is mixed in with the stools.

The diagnosis of piles may be obvious if they are visible around the opening to the anus. However, the doctor may insert a small instrument known as a proctoscope just inside the rectum to separate the bowel walls – a simple and painless procedure – to look for internal piles.

To relieve anal irritation due to piles, have daily warm salt baths and ask your pharmacist for a soothing emollient to apply. You may also need to use a course of suppositories (which contain an astringent to shrink the swollen inflamed tissue and a corticosteroid to reduce the inflammation) night and morning and after any bowel movement. It is also important to increase your intake of fluids and high-fibre foods, which, by helping to soften the stools, should reduce the need to strain or sit for long periods on the toilet.

If the symptoms do not improve, you may require surgery. This may involve injecting the swollen veins with a chemical which obliterates them; freezing them using a liquid nitrogen or carbon dioxide probe; or ligation, in which the base of each pile is tied off with a rubber band. In severe cases, surgical removal may be done under a general anaesthetic.

Pneumonia

Pneumonia is inflammation of the lungs, usually caused by a viral or bacterial infection, more rarely by a fungus or protozoa, and very occasionally brought on by accidental inhalation of vomit or a poisonous gas. The two main types are:

- **bronchopneumonia**, in which the infection starts in the bronchi and bronchioles (airways) before spreading to the surrounding lung tissue
- **lobar pneumonia**, in which the infection begins in a specific segment or lobe of one of the lungs.

Symptoms of pneumonia may include a cough that produces yellow or green sputum and occasionally blood, chest pains, breathlessness and fever. The severity of the illness will depend partly on the type of bug involved and partly on the general health of the person infected.

A diagnosis of pneumonia may be made from the symptoms, physical examination and chest X-ray. Although a sample of sputum may be sent to the laboratory to confirm the type of bug involved, the doctor may prescribe an antibiotic or anti-fungal drug immediately (depending on the suspected cause), as it can take several days for the results to be confirmed. In severe cases, treatment in hospital may be required, with oxygen therapy and even artificial ventilation if the person is struggling to breathe on his own.

In a healthy young adult, full recovery will usually take about two to three weeks, during which time the person will need to rest at home. In someone who already has respiratory problems, for example asthma or chronic bronchitis, pneumonia can be a lot more serious and potentially fatal. When pneumonia develops as a late complication of some other serious illness, such as stroke, cancer or AIDS, it may ultimately be the cause of death.

Pneumothorax

Pneumothorax is a condition in which air gets into the space between the inside of the chest cavity and the outer lining of one of the lungs. This air may enter the chest either from outside the body through a puncture wound in the chest wall or from a hole that suddenly and spontaneously appears in the lung itself.

A spontaneous pneumothorax is six times more common in men than in women. Typically, it occurs in thin, young, otherwise healthy adult men who have no apparent lung disease. However, it is believed that at least some of these men were born with a congenital blister at the top of the lung, which is more vulnerable to rupture.

Symptoms of a pneumothorax may include sudden onset of chest pain on the affected side and breathlessness, with the level of discomfort proportional to the amount of air pushing the lung to one side. If the pneumothorax continues to enlarge, to produce what is known as a tension pneumothorax, it may become life threatening by putting pressure on the heart.

A chest X-ray will usually be done to confirm the diagnosis. Treatment is not always necessary, because if the pneumothorax is small it will usually disappear on its own, with the air being reabsorbed over the next few days and any hole in the lining of the lung healing itself. However, a larger pneumothorax, or a small one in the presence of some underlying lung disease, may require a chest drain (insertion of a tube to release the trapped air and allow the lung to re-expand). If the lung fails to expand or if the pneumothorax recurs (of which there is about a 30 per cent chance), surgery may be required to seal the chest cavity.

Prostate enlargement

An enlarged prostate gland is a very common problem among older men. Each year in the UK, about 350,000 men visit their GP because of urinary symptoms due to an enlarged prostate, of whom about one in ten needs surgery. In almost all cases, the cause is benign prostatic hyperplasia (BPH) – a non-cancerous condition – hyperplasia meaning an increase in the number of cells within the prostate gland.

While it is normal for the prostate gland to enlarge around the time of puberty, as part of male sexual development, why it should start growing again in so many men once they pass the age of 50 is not understood. However, this renewed growth is known to be stimulated by dihydrotesterone, a breakdown product of testosterone – the male sex hormone produced by the testicles.

Because of the gland's position just underneath the bladder and surrounding the upper part of the urethra (the narrow tube that carries urine and semen to the tip of the penis), prostate enlargement may interfere with the normal flow of urine.

Until recently, the symptoms of BPH were attributed primarily to physical pressure exerted by the enlarged prostate gland on the urethra. However, it is now realised that symptoms are also the result of an increase in smooth muscle tone in both the prostate and neck of the bladder.

This explains why the severity of symptoms is not necessarily related to the size of the prostate gland. Minimal enlargement of the prostate may cause severe urinary symptoms that significantly disrupt daytime activities and interfere with sleep, while a large prostate may cause only minimal disability.

Characteristic symptoms of an enlarged prostate include:

- difficulty starting the flow of urine - you may have to push or strain
- a weak stream that may stop and start several times
- feeling that the bladder hasn't been completely emptied
- having to urinate again less than two hours later
- finding it difficult to postpone urination
- needing to urinate at intervals throughout the night
- dribbling after urination.

As a result of these symptoms, BPH may have a major impact on a man's quality of life. For example, he may have to restrict his intake of fluids before travelling anywhere or going to bed, be unable to drive far without a break, or go anywhere without toilets nearby, disturb his and his partner's sleep, or be embarrassed by episodes of incontinence.

Unfortunately, many men delay seeing a doctor until their symptoms have become intolerable, either because they are too embarrassed, or because they mistakenly think that their problem is an inevitable part of growing old. However, treatment nowadays, whether with drugs or surgery, is usually successful at restoring near-normal urinary function.

To confirm that the prostate gland is enlarged, the doctor may perform a digital rectal examination, whereby a lubricated gloved finger is inserted into the rectum and the prostate palpated (felt) through the front wall of the rectum, which lies against the back of the gland.

Most men suffering from BPH can now be effectively managed by drug treatment. The most effective type of drug prescribed is one of the selective alpha-1 blockers (tamsulosin, terazosin, doxazosin, alfuzosin, prazosin or indoramin), that can help relieve symptoms, not by altering the size of the gland, but by relaxing the smooth muscle inside the prostate and the neck of the bladder. The resultant reduction in pressure on the urethra can make it easier for the man to pass urine, relieving his symptoms and improving his urine flow as a result. Side effects from these drugs are usually minimal, although a few men complain of feeling dizzy and faint.

Another type of drug prescribed to treat BPH is the 5-alpha reductase inhibitor finasteride, which works by blocking the enzyme that converts testosterone to dihydrotestosterone, the hormone that stimulates the prostate to enlarge.

Treatment with finasteride can shrink the gland by as much as 20 per cent of its size over a 12-month period. However, the drug seems to only be effective in some men and can take at least six months to start to relieve symptoms.

Finasteride may also cause erectile dysfunction (impotence) and reduce libido in a few men. In addition, because finasteride passes from the man's circulation into his semen and may damage a developing foetus, condoms should be used during sexual intercourse if the man's partner is or may become pregnant.

If medical treatment doesn't provide sufficient symptom relief, there are severe symptoms, or if complications have developed, such as recurrent urine infection, bladder stones, retention of urine in the bladder or kidney damage resulting from back pressure, the man will usually be referred for a surgical procedure.

Surgery for BPH usually involves a trans-urethral resection of the prostate (TURP), in which a long narrow instrument (resectoscope) is passed up the urethra towards the bladder. At the tip of the resectoscope is an electrically heated wire loop that is used to shave away the obstructing prostate tissue, while the surgeon watches the procedure through a small telescope contained within the instrument.

TURP should make no difference to male libido, but it may occasionally cause impotence as a psychological response, particularly in men who haven't been properly counselled before their operation. A more common problem after TURP is retrograde (backward) ejaculation whereby, due to damage to an internal valve at the top of the urethra, semen is ejaculated back up into the bladder rather than out of the penis.

Retrograde ejaculation will cause the man to become infertile, although for most men old enough to require prostate surgery there is no desire to father a child. It should not make any difference to the enjoyment of sex, as long as both the man and his partner are aware of the reason why his orgasm is no longer producing a visible ejaculate.

Newer forms of surgical treatment, still under investigation as an alternative to conventional TURP, include the insertion of a tiny metal coil (stent) to open up the urethra inside the prostate, or the use of microwave or laser beams to destroy prostate tissue. If the prostate is very large, or there are bladder stones to be removed as well, an 'open' prostatectomy may need to be performed where the prostate is removed through an incision made in the lower abdominal wall. This operation requires a longer stay in hospital than transurethral surgery. It may also cause impotence and incontinence in some men and has been largely superseded by TURP.

Self-help measures for BPH that may reduce symptoms in less serious cases of prostate enlargement include:

- restricting fluid intake after 6pm
- cutting down on alcohol and caffeine
- limiting spicy food, which can further irritate the bladder
- taking exercise during the day if your lifestyle tends to be sedentary.

Prostatitis

Prostatitis is a condition in which the prostate gland becomes inflamed, usually due to a bacterial infection that has spread from the urethra. Occurring most commonly in men between the ages of 20 and 40 years, this infection may be sexually transmitted or develop as a complication of a urinary tract infection. Prostatitis in which no infection is found may be due to irritation of the prostate gland from the reflux of urine or as a result of tiny stones forming within the gland's ducts.

Symptoms of prostatitis may include pain or frequency passing urine, fever, low back pain, deep pain felt between the scrotum and anus, discharge from the penis and sometimes pain on ejaculation.

Diagnosis may be confirmed by rectal examination, in which the doctor inserts a lubricated, gloved finger into the rectum to feel the prostate gland through the front wall. The prostate will characteristically feel tender and swollen. To establish whether a particular bug is causing the inflammation, a sample of urine may be sent to the laboratory for analysis, along with a sample of urethral secretions, obtained after massaging the prostate gland during the rectal examination.

If prostatitis is due to a bacterial infection, treatment is with a prolonged course of antibiotics. Non-bacterial prostatitis may be treated with anti-inflammatory painkillers such as ibuprofen. Symptoms may persist for several months and also tend to recur.

Rashes

A rash is a group of spots or an area of abnormally red, flaky or scaly skin. Many rashes are only temporary and are not a sign of any skin disease or other medical disorder. A rash may:

- cover the whole body
- be localised to one area
- be accompanied by itching or by fever.

All the above symptoms can be clues to the underlying cause. Doctors also describe and assess a rash according to the types of spots that appear, for example papules are raised spots and macules are spots that are level with the surrounding skin but differ in colour or texture. In addition to assessing the types of spots, the distribution of the rash and the presence of any other symptoms, the doctor may carry out blood tests, take skin scrapings for examination under a microscope and/or examine the skin under a special lamp before making a diagnosis.

Treatment will then depend on the underlying cause, which might include any of the following conditions:

- **eczema/dermatitis** is characterised by a red, intensely itchy and scaly rash, which may occasionally weep. Treatment is with emollients and corticosteroid creams or ointments
- **psoriasis** causes areas of thickened inflamed blotches covered with silvery skin flakes. Treatment is with a range of creams and ointments containing vitamin D, coal tar, retinoids or corticosteroids; more severe cases may require drugs which suppress the immune system
- **rosacea** is associated with an abnormal redness of the face, particularly the nose and cheeks, accompanied by acne-like spots. Treatment is with antibiotic gel, tablets or capsules
- **urticaria** is a nettle rash with itchy white swellings which may develop as an allergic reaction to certain foods. Treatment is with antihistamines
- **prickly heat** causes intensely itchy red spots usually on the neck and front of the chest. Treatment is with antihistamines
- **fungal infections** such as ringworm (see page 269) may cause red scaly patches on the trunk or scalp. Treatment is with an antifungal drug
- **childhood infections** – a rash is the main sign of many common childhood illnesses, such as chickenpox, which causes red itchy spots that turn into blisters. Calamine lotion is still the most effective remedy to relieve the skin irritation caused by chickenpox
- **medical disorders** – an auto-immune disease such as rheumatoid arthritis or lupus erythematosus may cause a generalised rash, as well

as symptoms in other parts of the body. Treatment is with anti-inflammatory products and drugs which suppress the immune system

- **drug side-effect** – one common adverse reaction to many different types of drug is a generalised itchy skin rash.

Repetitive strain injury (RSI)

Any activity that involves repeating the same movement over and over again can result in damage to the parts of your body that are being overworked. This overuse injury, now more commonly referred to as repetitive strain injury or RSI, has received a lot more publicity over the last decade because of the epidemic of RSI among people who spend all day working on a word-processor.

Many supermarket checkout staff have also started to develop RSI since the introduction of the bar-code pricing system. To pass each individual item across the sensor, the same sweeping arm movement has to be performed hundreds of times each day. Other activities that can cause RSI include gardening, decorating and racquet sports such as tennis and squash.

Symptoms of RSI are typically pain and stiffness, which come on during the activity and ease off with rest. You may also feel numbness, tingling and swelling in the affected part. At first, you may notice only a mild discomfort that does not come on until you have been repeating the same movement for several hours and which goes away as soon as you stop. However, if you ignore or do not notice these warning symptoms, the condition is likely to deteriorate rapidly.

A few people with RSI have been forced to give up their jobs because of pain that comes on almost immediately they start work. Others are just about able to keep working but then have to put up with unpleasant symptoms for several hours afterwards.

Treatment for RSI may include applying an anti-inflammatory cream or taking anti-inflammatory painkillers. You may also be advised to rest the damaged tissues in a splint. Once the symptoms start to improve, you may be referred to a physiotherapist for a programme of exercises. Occasionally a corticosteroid injection into the painful area is required to relieve persistent inflammation.

To avoid RSI or to prevent a recurrence of this distressing problem, you should take the following steps:

- always work in a comfortable position
- try to relax when performing any repetitive task
- make sure your back and feet are well supported when you sit to work
- ideally your forearms should be pointing slightly downwards and your wrists should not be bent when you work for long periods with your hands
- take regular breaks during your working day
- do loosening up exercises after each work session
- never work through the warning symptoms of RSI
- make sure any instrument you are holding is the correct size, shape and weight for you
- check your technique with a more experienced colleague.

For an information pack, send a postal order or cheque for £3.95 made payable to the RSI Association.*

Rheumatoid arthritis

Rheumatoid arthritis (RA) is a severe form of arthritis that affects roughly one million people in the UK. The exact cause of RA is unknown, but it is believed to be an auto-immune disease, in which the body's immune system starts to attack its own tissues, in this case the joints. Although RA may begin at any age, it most commonly strikes people in their forties. In some cases, infection by a virus is thought to be the precipitating factor.

Symptoms of RA include:

- pain, tenderness, swelling, redness and warmth, usually affecting several joints symmetrically on either side of the body
- joint stiffness, characteristically worse on waking
- weakness of grip in one or both hands
- sometimes fever, malaise, general muscle weakness and weight loss.

These symptoms tend to flare up intermittently, with long periods of remission in between, which may last several months or even years. The diagnosis is made from a description of the symptoms and a physical examination of the inflamed joints. A blood test will usually show a high level of an abnormal protein known as rheumatoid factor.

Many RA sufferers only develop a mild disability and are able to remain mobile and independent. Treatment includes resting inflamed joints during a sudden flare-up, using splints, for example, and regular courses of physiotherapy at other times to loosen up the joints and strengthen the muscles that support them.

Non-steroidal anti-inflammatory drugs are prescribed to relieve the joint symptoms. In severe cases, drugs which slow down the disease and limit the amount of joint damage may be required – examples include gold salts, penicillamine and sulphasalazine – but all of these have potentially serious side-effects.

A variety of aids are available to help badly affected people overcome the disabling effects of RA, to cope with everyday tasks such as dressing and preparing food. Surgery may be necessary to correct a serious deformity, or to improve the range of movement in a joint.

Ringworm

Ringworm is the popular name for a group of common fungal infections of the feet, groin, trunk, scalp and nails, characterised by red, scaly skin, with or without blisters. The most common form of ringworm is athlete's foot (see pages 192–4), in which the fungus is picked up from damp floors or towels. With scalp and trunk ringworm, the fungi may be picked up from contact with an infected pet.

On the scalp, ringworm may lead to hair loss. On the trunk it is characterised by itchy patches that are circular and have a prominent edge. In the groin, ringworm (also known as jock itch) produces a red, itchy rash that may spread to the inside of the thigh; this type is much more common in men than women. When ringworm infects the toenails, as a complication of athlete's foot, they may become discoloured, thicken and start to crumble.

Although ringworm infections have a distinctive appearance, the doctor may want to confirm the presence of a fungal infection by examining skin scrapings under a microscope. Antifungal creams, ointments or lotions may be prescribed to treat ringworm of the skin. If the infection is severe or involves the hair or nails, you may have to take an anti-fungal drug by mouth. To ensure all the fungi are eradicated, treatment may need to be taken for some time after the symptoms have cleared up.

Salmonella

See 'Food poisoning'

Schizophrenia

Schizophrenia is a severe form of mental illness associated with delusions, hallucinations (usually hearing voices) and abnormal behaviour. It is sometimes referred to as having a 'split personality' because thoughts and feelings are no longer linked to each other in a logical fashion. Equally common in men and women, schizophrenia affects about one in every 100 people and usually comes on at some time between the ages of 15 and 30 years.

Symptoms may occasionally start suddenly in response to an episode of severe stress or after taking a mind-altering drug, but these factors are thought to unmask a mental illness that was already there, rather than be the underlying cause. Genetic factors are thought to play some role in the development of schizophrenia as this illness tends to be more common in certain families.

Often, the condition may pass unnoticed at first. The individual may simply become a little more withdrawn and introverted than before, or appear less motivated, which in an adolescent could easily be mistaken for a normal reaction to the emotional upheaval that commonly occurs at this time. It may only be once delusions or hallucinations start to obviously disturb a person's behaviour and thinking that the illness may begin to be recognised.

Schizophrenia can take many forms, for example the person may start to behave eccentrically or speak in a muddled and disjointed way, mixing up words and giving bizarre responses to questions. He may become paranoid, wrongly believing that someone is following him or trying to kill him. Another manifestation is catatonia, in which the individual performs strange, repetitive movements such as rocking, or adopts a rigid posture.

To make the diagnosis, the doctor will take a detailed history from the patient and his friends and family, looking for evidence of the characteristic symptoms and signs described above and also ruling out other mental illnesses such as depression and mania.

Treatment usually takes the form of anti-psychotic drugs, which may need to be given intermittently as a long-acting injection, combined with psychotherapy to help the individual understand and cope better with his illness. Unfortunately, although the drugs can be highly effective at suppressing psychotic symptoms, they may also be associated with unpleasant side-effects, such as abnormal muscle movements.

Some people with schizophrenia recover completely and never have another attack, others are able to lead relatively normal lives if they take their medication reliably, while a few require long-term hospital care. Unfortunately many of the schizophrenics who are discharged into community care are unable to cope, even with social service support, and end up in prison or living on the streets.

Sciatica

See 'Back pain'

Seasonal affective disorder

Seasonal affective disorder (SAD) is a type of depression that occurs during the winter months. In addition to making the sufferer feel low and miserable, possible symptoms include disturbed sleep, difficulty waking up in the morning or staying awake during the day, apathy, lethargy, fatigue, irritability, generalised aches and pains, reduced sex drive, loss of self-esteem and a craving for sugary foods which can lead to an unwanted increase in body weight.

As many as one in 20 people in the UK are thought to suffer from SAD each winter. The underlying cause is believed to be a biochemical imbalance in part of the brain known as the hypothalamus, brought on by a lack of exposure to natural sunlight.

If you have symptoms of SAD that have not been helped by spending more time exposed to natural daylight, then see your doctor. You may be referred to one of the specialist SAD clinics set up in different parts of the UK (contact SAD★ for details).

Treatment, which is successful in the majority of SAD sufferers, involves phototherapy – exposure to a very bright ultraviolet light, emitted from a light box that is at least ten times more intense than normal domestic lighting, for up to four hours a day. Occasionally, an antidepressant is also required.

Shingles

Shingles is a common viral infection caused by the same herpes zoster virus that causes chickenpox in childhood. Once the person has recovered from chickenpox, most of the viruses will have been destroyed. However, some remain dormant in the nerves, only to reappear as an attack of shingles many years later. Every year in the UK about one in 350 people develop shingles.

What actually triggers the virus to reactivate is unknown, but as the majority of sufferers are elderly, it may be the result of the immune system becoming less efficient as people get older. Occasionally, stress or being run down can bring on an attack of shingles by having a debilitating effect on the immune system. Drugs that are prescribed to suppress the immune system, for example to treat an auto-immune disease, and disorders that weaken the immune system such as AIDS can also bring on shingles.

The first warning symptoms of shingles may be either a severe burning discomfort in one specific part of the body, or the skin in that area becoming extremely sensitive. This may continue for several days until the distinctive rash appears. When the rash comes, it looks like chickenpox, with small raised red spots that turn into blisters. However, the rash covers only a strip of affected skin over the path of the affected nerve. Although the virus may strike anywhere, it is usually on one side of the chest, neck or face.

Antiviral drugs, such as aciclovir, valaciclovir and famciclovir, prescribed as soon as the rash first appears, can speed up recovery from shingles. These drugs also reduce the risk of developing the condition known as post-herpetic neuralgia, which is persistent pain in the affected nerve, due to damage from the virus, which may last for months or even years.

You may need to take anti-inflammatory painkillers for a few days to deaden the pain, and applying calamine lotion can ease any irritation from the rash. The blisters soon dry into scabs that fall off, and the rash will fade within two to three weeks. However, while the rash is visible, the virus is still contagious, and there is therefore a risk that you will give chickenpox to anyone with whom you come into contact (assuming they have not already had it).

When shingles involves the eye, emergency treatment from an eye specialist is essential to prevent permanent damage to the cornea at the front of the eye. If post-herpetic neuralgia does develop, a number of possible treatments can be given, including acupuncture, or an injection to deaden the damaged nerve.

Sinusitis

Sinusitis is a common condition in which the membranes lining the air-filled spaces (sinuses) in the front of the skull become inflamed. The usual reason for this inflammation is the spread of the viruses that cause the common cold from the nose into one or more of the surrounding sinuses.

In a healthy sinus, small amounts of mucus are produced which drain freely through narrow ducts into the nose. If a sinus becomes inflamed, much larger volumes of mucus are released. Although in many cases an episode of sinusitis will clear up without treatment after a few days – as the immune system kills off the viruses – occasionally it may result in a build up of mucus that is unable to drain away. Once fluid stagnates within the sinuses, there is then a risk of a secondary infection with bacteria that normally inhabit the nose and throat.

A persistent allergy may also cause sinusitis, as can any condition that interferes with sinus drainage, such as nasal polyps or deviation of the septum that divides the two nostrils. Infection from a tooth abscess may occasionally spread to involve the adjacent sinus.

Symptoms of sinusitis may include a congested feeling across the face, progressing to a severe throbbing pain, with swelling and tenderness over the affected sinuses. The person may also have a fever and feel dizzy and nauseous. Discomfort may be relieved by using a decongestant spray or drops or by inhaling vapours from a mixture of menthol and eucalyptus in hot water.

If your symptoms persist then seek medical help. Your doctor may arrange X-rays of the sinuses to determine the location and severity of the infection. If you have an underlying bacterial infection, a course of antibiotics will usually clear up the condition within a few days.

If the infection persists or is recurrent your sinuses may have to be washed out, using a warm, sterile salt solution flushed via a narrow tube pushed up the nostril and directly through the wall of the sinus. Any underlying cause will also need to be dealt with, for example removal of nasal polyps, or plastic surgery to straighten the nasal septum.

Snoring

Snoring is the noise made by vibrations in the roof of your mouth. It occurs most commonly in those people who breathe through their mouth while they are asleep, although it is also possible to snore through your nose with your mouth tightly shut.

Any condition which blocks the flow of air through the nose may produce snoring, for example a cold or sinus infection, a runny nose caused by allergy to dust, pollen or a particular food, polyps in one or both nostrils, a broken nose or enlarged adenoids. Your nose may also become blocked if the internal lining swells, which, apart from occurring as an allergic reaction, can happen as the result of stress, being overtired, smoking or eating a large meal.

Sleeping on your back increases the chance of snoring because this position encourages your tongue to slip to the back of your throat, partly blocking the air passages.

Simple home remedies for snoring include:

- losing excess weight
- sleeping in a more upright position, on pillows or by raising the head of the bed
- tying a scarf around the head and jaw to stop the mouth dropping open
- stitching a rolled-up sock or cotton reel to the back of the pyjama jacket (or nightgown) to make it too uncomfortable to sleep flat on your back
- putting a vaporiser in the bedroom, as a dry atmosphere encourages snoring
- cutting down on alcohol and not smoking
- avoiding late evening meals.

See your doctor if these measures don't make any difference, or if your partner has noticed that you regularly appear to stop breathing during the night as well – a condition known as sleep apnoea. The doctor may recommend a plastic device, now available in most large pharmacies, which, by widening the upper part of the nostrils, can improve air flow and stop snoring. A neck collar can help some snorers by keeping their lower jaw held forward while they sleep.

A surgical operation may be necessary if the underlying cause is a nasal polyp, enlarged adenoids, or if the septum inside the nose needs to be straightened. Steroid or decongestant nasal preparations may cure the problem if the nose becomes congested at night.

Spina bifida

Spina bifida is a congenital defect in which one or more of the vertebrae (spinal bones) fail to develop properly, leaving a section of the spinal cord exposed. This defect is usually in the lower back but can occur anywhere along the spine.

In the UK, about one in every 2,500 babies is born with spina bifida. The exact cause remains unknown, but the risk appears to be reduced if the mother takes a supplement of the vitamin folic acid from the time she starts trying to conceive until 12 weeks into the pregnancy. Once a couple has one child born with spina bifida, the chance of subsequent children being born with this condition increases.

There are four distinct forms of spina bifida. In one type, spina bifida occulta, the only defect is failure of the bony arches at the back of the spine to fuse. Occasionally, in this mild form, the spinal cord can become tethered to the defect, leading to problems with mobility and incontinence. However, in most cases, apart from a dimple or tuft of hair over the abnormality, the condition may pass unnoticed or be picked up only on a routine spine X-ray.

In the most severe form, myelomeningocele, the baby is born with a cystic swelling over the back; the swelling contains part of the spinal cord, which will either be damaged or not properly developed. As a result, the child will be seriously handicapped, with paralysis, loss of sensation below the level of the defect and incontinence. If this swelling contains only the meninges lining the spinal cord, known as a meningocele (the third form of spina bifida), then the nerves may have avoided being badly damaged, causing less disability as a result.

Finally, there is a rare disorder related to spina bifida in which the bones of the skull may fail to develop properly. If the cystic swelling that forms over the back of the skull, known as an encephalocele, contains part of the brain, the baby will usually be stillborn or die soon after birth.

Spina bifida may be diagnosed in early pregnancy from finding abnormally high levels of a substance known as alphafetoprotein in a routine antenatal blood test, or in the fluid removed during amniocentesis. A detailed ultrasound scan will then be carried out to establish the severity of the condition. The mother will then be given the option to have a termination.

A baby born with spina bifida may have surgery within the first few days of life to close the defect and prevent further damage to the spinal cord, although may still be left severely handicapped.

Most babies born with spina bifida also develop hydrocephalus, in which a blockage prevents cerebrospinal fluid draining normally from the ventricles (spaces) inside the brain down the spinal cord. This blockage is treated by the insertion of a shunt to draw off the excess fluid and prevent a dangerous rise in pressure inside the brain.

Modern surgical techniques, regular physiotherapy, training in self-insertion of a urinary catheter and good social service and educational support all contribute to helping all but the most severely affected children to lead productive and fulfilling lives. For further information, contact the Association for Spina Bifida and Hydrocephalus.*

Stroke

The overall incidence of stroke each year in the UK is about 200 victims for every 100,000 people. Older people have a much greater chance of suffering a stroke, with half the cases occurring in the over-75s.

A stroke is caused by interruption of the normal blood supply to part of the brain, resulting in damage to those brain cells deprived of oxygen for more than a few minutes. The three main types of stroke are: a cerebral thrombosis, in which a blood clot (thrombus) obstructs one of the main arteries in the brain; a cerebral embolism, whereby a fragment of blood clot that has broken off from elsewhere in the circulation blocks a brain artery; and a cerebral haemorrhage, caused by the rupturing of a blood vessel in the brain.

Symptoms of a stroke depend primarily on which part of the brain has been damaged, as each brain area controls specific functions related to particular parts of the body. Typical symptoms may include sudden onset of numbness or weakness, usually on one side of the body, loss of speech or slurring of words, a sudden severe headache, partial loss of vision, unexplained dizziness, confusion, a sudden fall or uncon-sciousness.

The diagnosis of a stroke is usually confirmed by a doctor carrying out a thorough physical examination. Occasionally, the extent of the brain damage may be assessed by a CT scan (a computer-generated cross-sectional X-ray) or some other brain-imaging technique.

If a stroke has been caused by a blood clot, drugs may be prescribed to dissolve the clot, to prevent the clot from enlarging, or to stop any further clots developing. A small daily dose of aspirin is commonly given to decrease the chance of a subsequent stroke. Only rarely is surgery performed to remove a blood clot or to stop bleeding from a ruptured artery.

The main element of stroke therapy is a rehabilitation programme that aims to improve physical abilities and restore independence. Although damaged nerve tissue will not regenerate, other parts of the brain may be trained to take over the functions of the damaged area.

Recovery is often a slow process and can be unpredictable. Although most of the improvement will occur in the initial few months, progress may continue to be made over several years. The success of stroke rehabilitation depends on the extent of brain damage, the skills of the various therapists involved, co-operation of family and friends and most importantly a positive attitude in the victim.

Measures to reduce the risk of stroke include:

- not smoking; limiting alcohol intake
- taking regular exercise
- eating a low-fat, high-fibre diet
- losing excess weight
- having regular blood pressure checks
- seeking medical attention if you suffer a TIA (see overleaf).

Subarachnoid haemorrhage

In this type of haemorrhage bleeding occurs over the surface of the brain between the middle and innermost membranes (meninges) that cover and protect the underlying nerve tissues. By contrast, when a stroke is caused by haemorrhage, the bleeding occurs within the brain itself.

Someone who suffers a subarachnoid haemorrhage typically develops a severe pain at the back of the head, which comes on suddenly and completely out of the blue, as if from a blow by a heavy object. The person will usually collapse and may lose consciousness for several hours or even days. The symptoms are similar to those of

TRANSIENT ISCHAEMIC ATTACK (TIA)

A TIA is a mini-stroke which causes symptoms similar to a normal stroke, but, because there is no permanent damage to the brain, these symptoms disappear completely within 24 hours, leaving behind no additional disability.

Typically, the victim of a TIA may suffer a sudden blackout, temporary loss of speech or vision, or transient loss of power or sensation in an arm or leg. Even though a full recovery may occur within minutes, it is still essential to see a doctor for a thorough check-up because a TIA is a warning signal that a major stroke could be on the way.

About 10 per cent of strokes are preceded by one or more TIAs, with the time delay varying from a few days to several months. Tests will usually be carried out to check the circulation to the brain, for example, an ultrasound scan of the arteries, or angiography, in which X-rays of the arteries are taken after a dye is injected into the circulation. A CT scan (computer-generated cross-sectional X-ray) of the brain may be done to rule out other brain disorders such as a tumour.

For some people who have had a TIA, the doctor may recommend aspirin or anticoagulant therapy, or surgery to remove fatty deposits from one of the arteries supplying blood to the brain as a way of reducing the chance of a future stroke.

meningitis – headache, vomiting, neck stiffness, a dislike of bright light and drowsiness.

Generally, the bleeding occurs spontaneously from a blood vessel at the base of the brain, which has ballooned due to a weakness in the artery wall that has been present since birth. Only a few cases are brought on by a head injury or strenuous physical exercise.

Subarachnoid haemorrhage can happen at any age, but is most common between the ages of 35 and 60. Diagnosis is confirmed if blood is found in a sample of spinal fluid drained from the lower back, along with a CT scan of the brain to locate the bleeding. Initial treatment, apart from bed rest, may include a drug to lower abnormally high blood pressure and a drug to relax spasm in the brain arteries.

Angiography – an X-ray of the brain arteries taken after injecting a dye, which shows up white on the subsequent pictures – may be carried out to see if surgical repair is feasible. Depending on the type of blood vessel damage and the severity of the haemorrhage, an operation may be performed to open the skull and clip the leaking blood vessel.

Alternatively, the vessel may be sealed using a special glue or metal coil, positioned using the angiography catheter (tubing) that is fed into a blood vessel in the brain via an artery in the groin.

Although subarachnoid haemorrhage may prove fatal, either at the time of the initial attack or due to subsequent bleeding, many victims recover – some completely, others with a residual disability such as limb weakness, memory loss or recurrent seizures.

Testicular disorders

A wide variety of disorders may affect one or both testicles. Cancer of the testicle has been discussed earlier in this chapter (see page 205). Some of the other more common testicular disorders are:

Undescended testicle   Occasionally, one or, even more rarely, both testicles fail to drop down into the scrotum. This condition occurs in about ten per cent of premature baby boys, but in only one per cent of boys born close to their expected date of delivery.

In many cases, the testicle descends on its own. However, if it doesn't come down within the first few months of life, surgical intervention is necessary. This operation, known as an orchidopexy, is usually performed before the age of five years to give the testicle a good chance of developing normally and also to reduce the risk of it failing to produce normal amounts of both sperm and testosterone in later life.

Retractile testicle   Another much more likely reason for one of the testicles appearing to be missing from the scrotum in a young boy is a condition known as a retractile testicle. Due to a powerful muscle reflex stimulated by cold or touch, the testicle is drawn up out of the scrotum into the groin. Careful examination by the doctor should distinguish a retractile from an undescended testicle.

Ectopic testicle   Here the testicle has migrated to an abnormal position, usually either in the groin or at the base of the penis, during development of the baby in his mother's womb. If this abnormality fails to correct itself spontaneously, surgery may be required to reposition the ectopic testicle in its rightful place.

Hydrocele   This is a collection of fluid in the scrotum which causes a soft painless swelling of the tissues surrounding one or both testicles. The cause in adults is usually unknown, although sometimes fluid is formed as the result of infection or injury.

Hydroceles occur most commonly in middle-aged men. Treatment is only necessary for a swelling large enough to be causing discomfort. Fluid may be drawn off using a sterile needle and syringe. However, if the hydrocele re-forms, surgery may be recommended.

Varicocele   This involves swelling of the veins above the testicle, most commonly just the left one. A varicocele is caused by a damaged valve in the vein draining blood from the testicle. This disorder is thought to affect as many as 15 per cent of adult men.

The aching discomfort sometimes caused by a varicocele may be relieved by wearing underpants that provide better support for the testicles. Surgery, carried out through a small incision in the groin, is reserved for those men whose discomfort persists, or cases in which the varicocele is thought to be interfering with sperm production, thus causing infertility.

Epididymal cyst   This is a fluid-filled swelling, usually painless, on the epididymis, which is the long coiled tube lying against the upper back part of the testicle, where sperm matures. This type of cyst is common in men over the age of 40 and surgical removal is necessary only if it becomes tender or enlarged.

Spermatocele   This harmless sperm- and fluid-filled swelling is also found on the epididymis. Again, surgical removal is necessary only if the swelling becomes large or uncomfortable.

Torsion of the testicle   Sudden severe pain and swelling of one of the testicles, sometimes with discolouration of the overlying scrotum and occasionally accompanied by abdominal pain and nausea, may be caused by the testicle twisting around in the scrotum, cutting off its blood supply.

Torsion occurs most commonly during puberty, although it can develop later. Emergency surgery is essential to prevent permanent damage to the testicle. The procedure involves untwisting the testicle and securing it in the scrotum with stitches.

If gangrene has already set in, the testicle will be removed, but as long as the other testicle is healthy, fertility should not be affected.

Orchitis   This is inflammation of one or both testicles causing severe pain and swelling, along with a fever. Orchitis may result from infection by the mumps virus, and about one-quarter of the few men who develop mumps after puberty suffer this complication.

Treatment is with painrelievers and icepacks, and symptoms usually settle down within a few days. Orchitis may cause the affected testicle to shrink, and can also interfere with fertility.

Epididymo-orchitis   In this condition, the testicle and its epididymis both become inflamed, usually due to a bacterial infection which in many cases has spread from the urinary tract. Symptoms include severe pain and swelling at the back of the testicle, accompanied by redness and swelling of the scrotum in some cases.

Because these symptoms can mimic a torsion of the testicle, surgical exploration may be necessary to confirm that the blood supply has not been obstructed. Treatment of epididymo-orchitis consists of bed rest and antibiotics. It may take several months for the testicle to return to its normal size.

Tinnitus

Tinnitus is a common condition in which noises are heard in one or both ears even though no such sounds are being made in the surrounding environment. This noise is usually a ringing sound, but it can also be whistling, buzzing, hissing or roaring.

Listening to loud music at a club or concert, or working with a power tool without wearing protective earplugs may cause tinnitus for several hours afterwards and indicates temporary damage to the hearing mechanism inside the inner ear. Repeated exposure to loud noises that cause this warning symptom may lead to permanent deafness later in life.

Minor causes of tinnitus include blockage of the ear canals with wax, a heavy cold that has resulted in congestion of the sinuses, or infection of the middle ear. Tinnitus may also occur as a side-effect of certain drugs, such as antibiotics, diuretics, quinine and high doses of aspirin.

Disorders of the inner ear, for example Meniere's disease, in which there is a build up of fluid pressure, and labyrinthitis, in which inflammation is usually due to a viral infection, are characterised by tinnitus accompanied by a disturbance of hearing and balance.

If you suffer from persistent or recurrent tinnitus you should be examined by a doctor because, in many cases, there is an underlying cause that will respond to treatment. However, if tinnitus remains a problem, many things can be done to make it more tolerable. For example, to mask the sound while reading or trying to fall asleep, you can listen to quiet music on the radio or ask your doctor about obtaining a tinnitus masker, which is worn like a hearing aid and provides more pleasant and less distracting sound.

Tonsillitis

Tonsillitis is an extremely common complaint among young children but may also occur infrequently in adolescents and young adults. The usual cause of tonsillitis is either a bacterial or viral infection.

During an attack of tonsillitis, one or both of the tonsils (oval-shaped spongy masses of lymph tissue located in the folds on either side of the back of the throat) become inflamed and swollen. This reaction is simply the result of the tonsils doing their job of protecting the body, particularly the upper part of the respiratory tract, against infection.

Each tonsil produces and stores millions of white blood cells capable of attacking the many different types of bug which may be inhaled through the mouth and nose. Inflammation and the formation of pus occur when the white blood cells inside the tonsils become activated and destroy the invading bugs.

Symptoms of tonsillitis may include sore throat, pain on swallowing, foul-smelling breath, tender swollen glands in the neck, headache and yellowish-white spots visible on the tonsils. Gargling with warm salt water can help to relieve the discomfort; paracetamol or ibuprofen can reduce the pain and fever. If the doctor thinks the infection is bacterial, he may take a throat swab to confirm the type of bug involved and prescribe a course of antibiotics.

Between infections, the inflammation and pus should disappear but it is perfectly normal for a child's tonsils to remain enlarged. The tonsils start to shrivel up once only a child passes the age of 10 years.

Unfortunately, in some children, the tonsils become overwhelmed by infection, so that instead of fighting off infections, they themselves become a focus for recurrent infection. As a result, the child may suffer repeated attacks of tonsillitis.

However, nowadays, doctors prefer to avoid surgically removing the tonsils if they can. The tonsils have an important job to do, and most children grow out of the problem. Surgery is usually done only if a child is missing an excessive number of days of school, if there is a complication such as an abscess on the tonsil or if an adult is suffering from recurrent tonsil infections.

Ulcerative colitis

Ulcerative colitis is a long-term condition in which the inner lining of the colon and rectum becomes inflamed. Although it may develop at any age, ulcerative colitis usually begins in early adulthood and is equally common in men and women. In the UK, ulcerative colitis currently affects about one in every 2,000 people.

Although the cause of the bowel inflammation is still unknown, it is thought that it may be an auto-immune disease, in which the body's immune system starts to attack its own tissues, in this case the large bowel.

Symptoms of ulcerative colitis may come on gradually, or begin as a severe attack of bloody diarrhoea, with frequent loose bowel movements containing pus, mucus and blood. Other symptoms may include abdominal pain, fever, loss of appetite and weight loss. About one in 10 of those affected just have one episode from which they recover completely and never have a recurrence. The remainder suffer intermittent attacks, usually with several months in between each.

In severe cases, ulcerative colitis can lead to anaemia as a result of excessive blood loss from the bowel, and inflammation may occur in other parts of the body, causing mouth ulceration, rashes, arthritis and painful red eyes.

Diagnosis can be confirmed using an endoscope (fibre-optic telescope which is passed up through the anus into the large bowel) and/or barium enema, which shows up areas of inflammation and ulceration in the bowel lining. Barium X-rays are usually not carried out during a flare-up because of the risk of perforating the acutely inflamed bowel wall. During endoscopy, a biopsy may be taken to provide a sample of tissue for examination under the microscope.

A bland low-fibre diet may help reduce the severity of symptoms during an attack. Drug treatment to control the inflammation may include corticosteroids given by mouth and sometimes as an enema; sulphasalazine; and other more powerful drugs which suppress the body's immune system.

Surgical removal of the colon may be necessary if the inflammation is extensive and cannot be controlled by drugs. If the rectum has to be removed as well, then the surgeon will create an ileostomy, which is an artificial opening in the abdominal wall through which bowel waste passes into a bag.

Because cancer of the colon occurs more commonly in people who have had ulcerative colitis for more than 10 years, regular screening by endoscopy may be recommended.

For more information, you should contact the National Association for Colitis and Crohn's disease.★

Varicose veins

Varicose veins are permanently enlarged, tortuous and twisted veins which may develop anywhere in the body but are found most commonly just under the skin surface in the legs. Examples of varicose veins in other parts of the body include piles (see pages 259–60) and a varicocele (see page 280). As many as 15 per cent of adults complain of at least some swelling of their leg veins; one in 100 are worried enough to visit a doctor because of them. Varicose veins are more common in some families than others, but other risk factors include:

- being overweight
- previous thrombosis in a leg vein
- standing for long periods in one position, for example working as a teacher.

Two main systems of veins in the legs carry blood back up towards the heart. The superficial veins, running just beneath the skin, take only about 10 per cent of the returning blood, and the deep veins that lie among the leg muscles shift the remaining 90 per cent. Blood is diverted from the superficial into the deep veins through a series of perforating veins.

In order to move blood against gravity back up the legs, the calf muscles act like a pump each time they contract. In addition, a series of one-way valves are positioned every few inches along both the deep and the perforating veins to prevent back flow.

Varicose veins appear when one or more of these valves become defective, with damage to one valve allowing blood to flow back and stretch the adjacent section of superficial vein. Failure of one valve also results in extra pressure on the next valve along, causing the condition to progress along the vein.

Many people with varicose veins have no symptoms, apart from the unsightly appearance of blue or purple swellings on one or both legs, which become more prominent if they stand for a long time. However, even mildly swollen veins can cause aching in the affected parts of the legs. This discomfort is due to stagnation of blood flow, which prevents the efficient removal of waste products from the surrounding tissues. In addition to aching legs, many sufferers are troubled by swelling of their feet and ankles, causing their shoes to feel tight by the end of the day.

If your varicose veins are causing increasing discomfort, ask your pharmacist or doctor for elastic support stockings. By squeezing blood from the superficial veins down into the deep veins, these stockings assist blood flow back up the leg and can ease your symptoms a great deal. Nowadays, a variety of support stockings specially designed for men are available; they look like ordinary socks where they appear below the hem of a pair of trousers. However, you will need to have measurements of your thigh, calf and ankle taken to ensure you receive the correct size so that the socks are comfortable and provide good support.

If you have just a few localised areas of swollen vein, the doctor may recommend sclerotherapy. In this procedure, pressure is put on the affected vein to empty it of blood, and then a strongly irritant solution is injected. The resultant inflammation shrivels up the inside of the vein forcing blood to be redirected to healthy veins. This treatment may need to be carried out over several sessions, with support stockings worn for a few days after each injection.

Surgical stripping of varicose veins may need to carried out if:

- you are unhappy about the cosmetic appearance of your legs
- you have persistent discomfort
- you have developed varicose eczema on your ankles
- you have suffered attacks of phlebitis (inflammation of the leg veins)
- the veins are now large enough to risk haemorrhage if they were knocked.

If you have bad varicose veins, you need to take extra care of the skin on your legs. Because of the stagnated blood flow, some parts of the skin may become deprived of oxygen, resulting in patches of inflammation and a risk of ulceration. To protect your skin, use a moisturiser on any dry patches, try to avoid unnecessary knocks or scratches, do not warm your legs in front of the fire or on a hot water bottle, and apply a sunscreen when you are out in the sun. To help prevent varicose veins, or to ease your symptoms if you already have them:

- never cross your legs or ankles when either sitting or standing
- if you sit or stand for a long time, do some foot and ankle movements to get the blood flowing
- at the end of the day, sit or lie with your feet raised above your hips
- avoid tight socks or garters
- do regular leg exercises
- keep your weight within normal limits
- if you smoke, stop or cut down because nicotine further interferes with blood flow and carbon monoxide in inhaled smoke further reduces the supply of oxygen to your tissues
- consider raising the foot of the bed with two inch blocks.

Verruca

A verruca (plantar wart) is a wart that grows on the sole of the foot. The highly infectious wart virus that causes a verruca may be shed on to a floor, where it may be picked up by another bare foot. It is thought that the virus enters the skin through a tiny crack, and this is more likely to happen when the foot is wet or sweaty, for example when a person is walking barefoot at the gym, swimming-pool or in a changing room.

It is easy to mistake a verruca for a splinter because typically it has a tiny black or brown pinpoint at its centre. However, a verruca will normally have several of these points, and the surrounding skin will feel rough and be irregular in shape.

Unlike most types of wart, which are not painful, a verruca often becomes sore and tender because it is pressed up into the sole of the foot each time weight is put on it. Nowadays, the doctor may decide not to treat a verruca because this type of wart usually goes away by itself. Also, if it is removed too soon, the person will not have time to build up natural immunity, and therefore is at risk of picking up another verruca in the future.

If the verruca is causing you a lot of pain, then your doctor may prescribe salicylic acid gel (which dissolves the top layers of skin), to be applied once daily. Before each treatment, you should sand off the upper layers of dead skin using an emery board. Then after soaking the foot in warm water to soften the skin, apply the gel, taking care not to put it on surrounding healthy skin.

Using a foam pad with a central hole positioned over the verruca is a good way to ease the discomfort while the verruca is being treated. If the verruca persists, then you may need to have it burnt off using a liquid nitrogen probe or laser treatment, which can take two or three treatments.

Warts

Warts are very common, contagious but harmless skin growths which may appear on almost any part of the body. They are caused by the human papilloma virus, and there are over 30 different types, of which just some are responsible for specific types of wart at specific sites in the body.

Warts are spread by direct contact and it is possible to spread a wart from one part of your body to another. It may take any time up to 12 months for a wart to appear after being infected. The wart virus only affects the top layers of the skin. The black dots that sometimes appear are tiny blood vessels that become clotted.

- **Common** warts are well defined, raised, rough-textured growths that often appear in clusters and vary in colour from grey to yellow or brown. Some are barely visible, while others grow to over 2cm across. They typically appear on areas of skin prone to injury, such as the hands and knees.
- **Flat warts** are smooth, slightly elevated growths that are flesh or tan coloured and may itch. They occur mainly on the face, wrists and backs of the hands, or along the line of a scratch.
- **Filiform warts** are long, frond-like growths that may appear on the eyelids, in the armpits and on the neck.
- **Digitate warts** have finger-like projections and are sometimes dark in colour.
- **A plantar wart**, found on the sole of the foot, is popularly referred to as a verruca (see page 286).

- **Genital warts** are a type of sexually transmitted disease (see pages 123–4).

About half of all warts will disappear within 12 months without treatment, which is why warts other than genital warts are often left to disappear naturally. Unsightly warts, or those that persist, may be treated with salicylic acid gel, which dissolves the top layers of skin, or burnt off using a liquid nitrogen probe or laser treatment.

Appendix I

Making the most of your doctor

You can make the experience of visiting your GP more rewarding and less stressful by following the advice given below. You should not worry about wasting your doctor's time with something trivial; it will not take long for him to reassure you if nothing is seriously wrong with you. It is important that you do not put off going because you are afraid you will be given bad news as the earlier a diagnosis can be made, the more straightforward and successful your treatment is likely to be.

When you make an appointment, you will need to tell the receptionist a little about your problem so that he or she can decide how quickly you need to be seen. The information you give will be treated in complete confidence. Do not believe the popular myth that all receptionists are dragons – most are polite and helpful and will make sure that you see your doctor as quickly as is necessary. However, if you do have any difficulty, let your doctor know.

It is always best to try to visit your usual doctor, especially if you are already receiving treatment or if you are returning with a problem that has not cleared up. You will usually be able to choose whether you see a male or female doctor, but remember that female doctors do not get embarrassed easily and should be as sympathetic and understanding as a male doctor, whatever your problem.

At the start of the consultation, your doctor will want to know what your main symptoms are, when they started and how they have changed. You may be asked to explain exactly what you mean when you are describing your symptoms; do not be offended by this because symptoms such as indigestion, for example, mean different things to different people, and your doctor will want to be sure exactly what you are complaining of. Be prepared to answer questions that might seem irrelevant to you, for example, if you say you have a pain, you will usually be asked to describe what it feels like, as this can provide important clues to the diagnosis.

Do not exaggerate or interpret your symptoms; just use your own words and let your doctor decide how serious they are. You may find it helpful to write a brief summary of what you want to say before your visit so that you do not worry about leaving out anything important.

Patients often complain that their doctor does not explain what is going on, but this may be because he or she thinks you already know or perhaps used language you didn't understand. Don't be afraid to ask questions, such as how long your symptoms are likely to last and whether there is anything you should or should not do. To help you remember what you are told, it may be worth taking a few notes, which you can look at later. Remember that your doctor will not always have all the answers; it may be necessary to wait for the results of tests or to see how things develop, and sometimes you may get better before a diagnosis has been made.

If you are given a prescription, you should ask what it is for and make sure you know how to take it and which side-effects to report. If you are unhappy about taking the treatment, say so at the time to give your doctor the chance to reassure you. However, you should not always expect a prescription, as many minor illnesses get better without treatment.

Don't be afraid to telephone your doctor for advice. You should try to ring during surgery hours so that you can speak to a doctor who knows you. The best time to ring is at the end of morning surgery, unless you think you might need a visit, in which case you should ring as soon as the surgery opens – this allows your doctor time to plan the visits for that day. Before you ring, make a list of the questions you want to ask so you do not forget anything. One important question to ask is when to call again if your symptoms have not improved.

Referral for hospital treatment

From time to time, you may need to be referred to the outpatient department of your local NHS hospital. According to the Patient's Charter (see pages 293–5), you should be seen in the outpatient clinic within 26 weeks of referral (the standard the Charter has set for hospitals is that 9 out of 10 patients should be seen within 13 weeks). The hospital will write to you with details of your appointment. Also according to the Charter, when you attend the outpatient clinic you should be seen within 30 minutes of your appointment time.

If you are about to be admitted to hospital as an inpatient, for example to have an operation, discuss with your GP the nature of the procedure and the possibility of other treatment options. It is also advisable to have the same discussion with the surgeon. If you are worried, or feel you have not been given enough information, you are entitled to ask for a second opinion.

Under the Patient's Charter, you should be given, before or at the time of admission, a written and a verbal explanation of what will happen during your hospital stay. Before any surgical procedure takes place, you will be asked to sign a consent form. First, be sure that you know the answers to all of the following questions:

- what is the reason for the operation?
- what is going to be done and what are the risks?
- who will perform the operation and how much experience does he or she have of this procedure?
- how long will I be in hospital?
- how long will it take me to recover?
- will I be in pain afterwards, and if so what pain relief will be available?
- are there likely to be any permanent after-effects?

Changing your doctor

To get the best out of your doctor you need to have confidence in his or her ability and trust his or her judgement. If you are unhappy or feel uncomfortable with your present doctor, or if there is a clash of personality between you, it is not difficult to change and you do not have to give a reason. However, it is worth making an appointment first to talk things through to give your doctor a chance to improve matters. If you feel you want a second opinion, most doctors will be happy to refer you to a specialist. As a last resort you can change to a new doctor. Another reason why you might have to change your doctor is if you move out of the practice area.

Once you have decided to change your doctor, all you have to do is go to the surgery of your choice in your area and ask to be registered. You do not have to ask your current doctor for permission to change or ask him or her to sign the back of your medical card. You also don't have to give a reason.

Nowadays, it is supposed to be easier than in the past to transfer to a new doctor. However, in a few rural areas, where there might be only one practice, or even only one doctor for miles around, your freedom of choice is limited. In addition, a doctor can refuse to let you join his practice without giving you a reason. No doctor is obliged to take you on as a patient unless you have been unable to find any doctor in your area prepared to accept you voluntarily; if this happens, you will be allocated to a particular GP by your local Family Health Services Authority (FHSA).

Although most people have no problem joining their doctor or practice of choice, difficulties can arise if:

- the doctor's list is full; a maximum list size is recommended for each GP
- you live outside the practice area; in the event of needing an emergency visit, it would take the doctor longer to travel from your home to any subsequent emergency call
- you are likely to need a lot of medical care, such as regular home visits; some elderly, disabled or chronically ill patients have found it extremely difficult to change their doctor.

What do you want from your doctor?

Assuming a selection of practices are prepared to put you on their books, here is a checklist of questions to consider when choosing a new GP:

- do you need the surgery to be within walking distance, on a bus route or just accessible by car?
- how flexible are the surgery hours; can you have an appointment outside your normal working hours?
- does the surgery have an appointments system or are you seen on a first-come-first-served basis?
- if it is difficult for you to use a telephone while you are working, does the surgery take phone calls for appointments and enquiries during the lunch hour?
- would you be able to see your doctor on most days of the week or is he or she unavailable on some days?
- would you have the freedom to see any of the doctors working in a group practice?

- does the surgery offer speciality services, such as men's health, sports injuries, counselling or complementary therapy clinics?
- if you are planning a family, does the practice offer shared antenatal care with the local consultant, thereby reducing the number of hospital visits for your partner?
- would you have direct access to the practice nurse to deal with minor health problems?
- are minor operations performed at the surgery, saving a long wait for a hospital appointment?

Choosing a new doctor

When you are looking for a new GP, ask your FHSA whether a directory of the local practices – giving details about each of their doctors and the services they offer – has been produced. Most surgeries now provide their own information leaflet for prospective patients as well as people already registered with them.

You will also be able to find a list of the GPs practising in your area in your local Post Office, Citizens' Advice Bureau and public library. In addition, it is worth seeking the opinion of friends and neighbours; and why not visit the surgery or health centre to inspect the facilities and talk to the receptionists?

If you are changing to another doctor in the same area because of a dispute, it is probably wise to choose one from a different practice and one that does not share the same on-call rota with your old doctor. Otherwise, you run the risk of having to see your original doctor when your new one is unavailable.

When you change, it is important to remember that although your new medical card should arrive within a few days of filling in a registration slip at the surgery or completing part A of your previous medical card, your medical records can take many months to be transferred. Occasionally, they even get lost in transit. Therefore, it is advisable to take a summary letter from your last doctor, especially if you are currently under any treatment.

What are your rights as a patient?

The Patient's Charter, launched in 1991 and extended several times since, sets out the rights and standards that you can expect throughout the NHS. Your rights under it are:

- to receive healthcare on the basis of clinical need, regardless of ability to pay
- to be registered with a GP
- to be able to change doctors easily and quickly
- to be offered a health check on first joining a doctor's list
- to receive emergency medical treatment at any time through a family practitioner, the emergency ambulance service and hospital accident and emergency department
- to have appropriate drugs and medicines prescribed and to have any proposed treatment clearly explained to you, including any risks involved and any alternatives
- to be referred to a consultant acceptable to you when your GP thinks it necessary and to be referred for a second opinion if you and your GP agree that this is desirable
- to have access to your health records (post 1991) and to know that those working for the NHS are under a legal duty to keep their contents confidential
- to choose whether or not to take part in medical research or medical student training
- if aged between 16 and 74 and not seen by your doctor in the previous three years to have the health check to which you are entitled under the existing health promotion arrangements; and to be offered an annual health check (at home if you wish) if 75 years old or over
- to be given detailed information about local family doctor services, including quality standards and waiting times, through your health authority/board's local directory
- to receive a copy of your doctor's practice leaflet, setting out the services he or she provides
- to receive a full and prompt reply to any complaints you make about NHS services
- to be guaranteed admission for virtually all treatments by a specific date no later than 18 months from the day when your consultant places you on a waiting list.

The Patient's Charter is to be replaced in 1999 with a new NHS Charter, which will set standards of care you can expect but will also state what the NHS can expect from you, i.e. your responsibilities. Patients will have to keep, or call to cancel, appointments, think twice before calling out a GP to their home and treat NHS staff with respect. This change in emphasis should help to further improve the relationship between you (the patient) and your doctor.

Making a complaint

If you want to complain about your GP:

- telephone or write to your local FHSA within 13 weeks of the incident that has upset you
- minor complaints, such as rudeness, may be dealt with informally by the FSHA
- a more serious allegation, for example refusing to visit, can result in a service committee hearing in front of lay and professional members appointed by the FHSA. You may be asked to attend and give evidence. This committee can recommend that the offending GP be given either a warning as to his or her future conduct or a financial penalty
- if you think your doctor has behaved unethically or unprofessionally, for example through drunkenness, sexual impropriety or disclosing confidential medical information, you should complain directly to the General Medical Council★
- for further advice and assistance in making a complaint against your GP, contact your local Community Health Council – the telephone number can be found in the phone book
- if you are seeking financial compensation, you will usually have to take legal action and prove negligence in court. In some cases, a hospital trust or health authority will settle out of court in the form of an ex gratia payment, as a goodwill gesture rather than through any legal obligation. It is essential to take legal advice from a lawyer with experience in medical negligence. For more information and names of suitable lawyers in your area, contact Action for Victims of Medical Accidents★
- if you remain unhappy about the outcome of your complaint, you can appeal to the Ombudsman (Health Service Commissioner), who is independent of the NHS and the Department of Health. You will need to put your complaint in writing within one year of the event. If the Ombudsman decides you have a case, he or she has right of access to all your NHS records as part of his or her investigation.

Men's health on the Net

Thousands of people in the UK regularly access the Internet to find information about a wide variety of different health topics. However, once you start 'surfing' the Net, you will soon discover that each health keyword you type into a search engine will produce a list of hundreds of web sites for you to choose from. So how can you sort out which sites contain accurate and reliable medical information and which are promoting highly dubious 'miracle cures' and 'magic remedies', for which there is actually no scientific proof that they work? For example, after the US Food and Drug Administration approved Viagra for the treatment of erectile dysfunction, several web sites appeared on the Internet, providing information about the benefits of Viagra, but selling products with similar names such as 'Viagro' and 'Vaegra'; in reality, these products were nothing more than herbal supplements. It was only when Pfizer, the pharmaceutical company that manufactures Viagra, began filing lawsuits that these web sites disappeared.

Rather than using the more popular search engines, Robert Kiley, writing in the *Journal of the Royal Society of Medicine* in July 1998, recommends using a 'quality search filter'. The Health on the Net Foundation (www.hon.ch/), for example, includes only those web sites written by medically/health trained and qualified professionals, and if it includes ones that are written by anyone else, then there has to be a disclaimer saying that 'the piece of advice offered is from a non-medically/health qualified individual or organisation'.

When you are accessing a web site, ask yourself the following questions to help assess the credibility of the information you are reading:

- are the authors of the text clearly stated and, if so, are their qualifications listed?
- is the name of the organisation that developed the web site displayed and are there any sponsors or advertisers who may have unduly influenced the messages within an article?
- are any statements about the effectiveness and safety of a product backed up by scientific data from a medical journal?
- has the web site been updated recently?

You also need to be careful when you follow a hypertext link, which may take you away from a good quality site to one where the information is misleading or medically inaccurate.

I have reviewed the following mixture of men's health web sites, almost all of which derive from the USA. Some of them are magazine-style sites that have been written by medical journalists, rather than physicians. However, they are still informative, and when I accessed them at the time of writing, they appeared to be of good quality.

The key point to bear in mind before you check out any of these sites is that they are designed for information purposes only. They should certainly not be relied upon for diagnosis or treatment and they are not designed to replace advice and care from your general practitioner.

Web sites

malehealthinstitute.com
Web site created by Dr Ken Goldberg, the founder of the first US centre specialising in male health; topics include common men's health problems and symptoms, self care and sexual health.

www.malehealthinstitute.com/colindex.html#anchor41026257
An A–Z list of articles written by the founder of the US-based male health institute, Dr Ken Goldberg.

www.sleh.com/healthservices/menshealth.htm
Information in the form of factsheets on a variety of men's health topics, with a comprehensive section on male reproductive health, produced in the USA from St Luke's Episcopal Hospital, University of Texas.

www.jeffersonhealth.org/diseases/mens_health/toc.htm
A wide range of men's health topics are covered in detail in the form
of news stories, feature articles and educational information on specific
disorders. This web site is produced by the Jefferson Health System, a
US healthcare organisation that provides a network of hospitals, clinics
and other health services to patients in the Philadelphia region.

www.healthtouch.com/level1/leaflets/101529/101529.htm
Part of a larger web site produced by the US-based company Medical
Strategies Inc. ('Online for better health'); topics covered include heart
disease and stroke; sexual and reproductive health; men and cancer;
men's mental health and physical addictions; kidney, urological and
sexual problems; benign prostatic hyperplasia and other prostate
problems; nutrition and staying healthy. Information is endorsed by
US-based professional associations.

www.impotencepartnerships.com
Site developed for an international audience containing distinct
sections for patients, partners, and a password-protected section for
physicians; content, which includes a patient questionnaire –
'impotence-could this be you?' – is approved by an independent panel
of experts. The site is supported by an educational grant from Astra
Pharmaceuticals.

www.prostate.org/index.html
Educational site for people suffering from prostatitis (inflammation of
the prostate gland), produced as an official communication of the US-
based patient group the Prostatitis Foundation.

www.mit.edu/afs/athena/user/p/a/pandre/www/Cancer.html
Web site developed by the Massachusetts Institute of Technology in the
USA; provides information on all aspects of cancer, including the
emotional and economic impact on the individual; targeted at US
cancer sufferers but still useful for UK readers.

www.tinactin.com/frameset.html
Information on prevention and treatment of common sports injuries,
plus training tips for a variety of sports, written by US specialist Mr Mark
Smaha, Director of Athletic Medicine, Washington State University; site

sponsored by US pharmaceutical company Schering Plough to advertise its antifungal treatment for athlete's foot, jock itch and ringworm.

www.plainsense.com/Health/Mens/
US site covering a long A–Z list of men's health problems from athlete's foot to weight control; information does not seem to be endorsed by any specific physician or professional organisation, but it does seem to be both trustworthy and useful. Each topic includes a 'When to see a doctor' section.

www.yt.sympatico.ca/Contents/Health/health.html
Canadian web site covering all aspects of health, with a special section devoted to the 'men's health community'; in addition to articles on physical, emotional and sexual health, topics include how to get the most from your doctor and reviews by doctors of new drugs just launched in Canada.

www.mediconsult.com/men/
US site containing a mixture of medical news, plus links to educational sites on a range of health topics of relevance to men; supported by advertising of US health products.

www.vix.com/menmag/mensheal.htm
In addition to covering common men's health problems, such as male menopause, testicular cancer and hair loss, this US site covers male role/responsibility topics such as fatherhood and gender issues; also advertises a number of men's health publications.

www.menshealth.com/index.html
Magazine-style site, again from the USA. Contains information about men's lifestyle (it is not a health guide). However, it does include tips on diet, exercise, and answers readers' health queries.

www.betterhealth.com/HK/SubjectMain/0,1344,180,00.html
Another magazine-type site from the USA; in addition to a range of men's health topics, this site gives free access to Medline (a database of medical papers on any topic) and AIDSLine (a database of medical papers on AIDS-related subjects), plus the opportunity to join message groups on prostate cancer and general men's health topics.

www.mensfitness.com/
Magazine-style site, produced by the US publisher of *Men's Fitness*; its target audience is young active males. The site covers fitness, health, nutrition, lifestyle and sexual issues.

Glossary

abscess A localised collection of pus that forms as a result of infection, usually involving bacteria, sometimes fungi or amoebae. Pus contains the infecting bugs (dead and alive), white blood cells that have been drawn to the area to fight the infection, and tissue cells that have been damaged by the infection. Because a lining usually surrounds the abscess, which reduces the amount of drug that can reach it from the bloodstream, treatment involving surgical drainage may be required

acid reflux A backflow of stomach acids (which aid the digestion of food) into the oesophagus (gullet) causing heartburn. Acid reflux may occur when the muscular valve around the lower end of the oesophagus – which normally prevents these acids escaping from the stomach – is put under too much pressure, for example from being overweight or from overeating. The cause may also be a weakness of this valve associated with a hiatus hernia (where part of the stomach protrudes upwards into the chest cavity through the diaphragm)

acute Sudden onset

addiction The need to use repeatedly a drug, such as nicotine, alcohol or heroin. Addiction (or dependence) can be physiological, in which case stopping the drug will cause unpleasant withdrawal symptoms, and/or psychological, with intense craving if the individual is deprived of the drug

adenoids Lymph tissue in the form of swellings at the back of the nasal passages, which form part of the body's defence system, helping to prevent the spread of infections from the nose to the throat and the rest of the upper respiratory tract. The adenoids tend to enlarge during early childhood in response to repeated infections but start to shrink after the age of six or seven, disappearing altogether at puberty. If they remain abnormally large in late childhood, blocking the flow of secretions to cause recurrent middle ear or sinus infections, surgical removal may be advised

adrenaline A hormone released by the adrenal glands in response to stress, fear, anxiety or exercise which stimulates a variety of changes inside the body, including an increase in the heart and breathing rates, diversion of blood from the digestive system to the muscles and a rise in blood sugar levels, all of which increase the body's physical efficiency

AIDS (Acquired Immune Deficiency Syndrome) A condition which develops as a result of infection with the Human Immunodeficiency Virus (HIV, see page 308). AIDS may result in a variety of diseases, most of which are due to the virus causing failure of the body's immune defences against infection and cancer

amino acids Chemical building blocks from which proteins are made that each contain carbon, nitrogen and oxygen. Each protein in the body contains up to 20 different amino acids linked together in long folded chains in a specific sequence

anaemia A condition in which the oxygen-carrying pigment, haemoglobin, within the red blood cells is reduced in concentration. There are many causes, including lack of iron (an essential ingredient of haemoglobin), excessive destruction of red blood cells and reduced production of new red blood cells in the bone marrow, caused by certain types of drugs and viral infections. Because haemoglobin is responsible for carrying oxygen from the lungs to the body tissues, symptoms of anaemia will be due to a lack of oxygen reaching different parts of the body. These symptoms may include tiredness, breathlessness, dizziness and chest pain. The lower the concentration of haemoglobin, the worse the symptoms – although some people with long-term anaemia may adapt to this oxygen deficiency

angioplasty A surgical technique to improve blood flow through an artery narrowed by disease. An inflatable balloon and/or powerful laser beam may be used to widen (or re-open) the narrowed (or blocked) section of the artery

antenatal Occurring before birth

antibiotic Any one of a variety of drugs that can kill or stop the growth and proliferation of bacteria inside the body. Originally derived from moulds and other living micro-organisms, nowadays the majority of antibiotics are made artificially from chemical ingredients

antibodies Proteins produced by lymphocytes (a type of white blood cell) in response to contact with an antigen (see below), which either neutralise the antigen or make it more vulnerable to destruction by other white blood cells

antigen Any substance recognised by the body as being foreign. An antigen causes the body's immune system to produce antibodies (see above) which neutralise or destroy it. Although antigens are usually proteins (such as parts of viruses, bacteria, fungi, pollen, dust mite faeces or a donated organ), other substances such as metal may have an antigenic effect by combining with and modifying one of the body's own proteins

antihistamine A type of drug which blocks some of the actions of histamine (a body chemical which irritates and inflames tissues causing an allergic reaction, such as hay fever)

artery A tube with elastic, muscular walls which carries blood away from the heart

auto-immune disease A group of diseases, all of which occur as a result of the body's immune system (natural defences) attacking its own organs and tissues. Normally the immune system only targets foreign material such as cancer cells or invading bacteria or viruses. Auto-immune diseases include rheumatoid arthritis (see pages 268–9) and insulin-dependent diabetes mellitus (see pages 218–20).

basal metabolic rate The amount of energy (Calories, see overleaf) consumed by the body at rest to maintain vital functions such as heartbeat, breathing and digestion

beta-blocker A drug which prevents the stimulation of body organs, tissues and vessels both by sympathetic nerves and by adrenaline (see page 302) in the bloodstream. Betablockers may be prescribed to relieve symptoms of anxiety or an over-active thyroid gland, to prevent migraine attacks or angina, to lower high blood pressure, or to control abnormal heart rhythms

bile The thick greenish-brown fluid which is formed in the liver from broken-down red blood cells and other waste products; it is stored and concentrated in the gall bladder and released intermittently into the duodenum to help with the digestion of fats

blackhead A type of spot characteristically seen on the surface of the skin of acne sufferers

bypass surgery A procedure to restore the normal flow of blood, urine, intestinal contents or spinal fluid around a blockage which has developed in part of the body. Coronary artery bypass surgery – one of the most commonly performed bypass operations – is often effective in relieving angina or preventing a heart attack in men with obstructed arteries in their heart circulation

Calorie The unit used to measure the energy value of food and drinks. One Calorie (kilocalorie) represents the amount of heat required to raise the temperature of one kilogram of water by one degree centigrade

capillary The smallest type of blood vessel in the body. Networks of capillaries around the body receive blood from arteries and drain blood back into the veins. Because the capillary wall is only one cell thick it allows a free exchange of oxygen, nutrients, salts, water, carbon dioxide and other waste products between the bloodstream and surrounding tissues

carbohydrate The body's main source of food energy, carbohydrates are made up of saccharide molecules, which each contain carbon, hydrogen and oxygen. Simple carbohydrates (sugars) cause a sharp rise in blood sugar and include sucrose (cane or beet sugar), fructose (fruit or honey sugar) and lactose (milk sugar). Complex carbohydrates (starches) have to be broken down in the digestive system before they can be absorbed, thus producing a steady, more prolonged rise in blood sugar levels. Starches are found in fruits, vegetables, wholegrain breads, cereals and pasta. A refined carbohydrate is one which has been processed, for example white sugar or polished rice, lowering its fibre content and reducing slightly its vitamin and mineral levels

cartilage Dense connective tissue capable of withstanding considerable pressure. Different types of cartilage perform different functions throughout the body; elastic cartilage, for example, provides the framework for the outer part of the ear; disks of fibrous cartilage act as shock absorbers between the vertebrae and inside the knee

chemotherapy The use of one or more chemical substances to prevent or treat disease; the term is used most commonly to describe treatment prescribed to people with cancer, either to shrink a tumour or to reduce the chance of it spreading to other parts of the body

chest infection A popular term for two different types of lower respiratory tract infection: bronchitis (see pages 198–9) and pneumonia (see pages 260–1).

cholesterol A chemical found in the bloodstream and body tissues which is a key component of cell membranes and a vital ingredient of steroid hormones, including testosterone. Most cholesterol is produced by the liver when it processes digested saturated fat – only a small amount comes directly from cholesterol-containing foods, such as eggs and some types of shellfish. Abnormally high amounts of cholesterol in the bloodstream increase the risk of a heart attack or stroke

chronic Persistent

cirrhosis Scarring inside the liver as a result of its cells being damaged, for example through excessive alcohol consumption, or infection with hepatitis B

colitis Inflammation of the colon, which may cause severe diarrhoea, blood or mucus in the faeces, pains in the lower abdomen and, sometimes, fever. Colitis may be due to a bacterial infection, amoebic dysentery or inflammatory bowel diseases, such as Crohn's disease (see pages 212–13) or ulcerative colitis (see pages 283–4)

colostomy A surgical procedure whereby the cut end of the colon is brought through the muscles at the front of the abdominal wall to form a new opening (stoma) from which faeces can be evacuated into a disposable waterproof bag attached to the surrounding skin. A colostomy may be a temporary measure (to allow the bowel to heal after an operation) or a permanent one (if the rectum has had to be removed)

coronary thrombosis A medical term for a heart attack in which one of the heart arteries is obstructed by a clot. This results in death of the heart muscle because it does not receive the vital oxygen and nutrients normally provided by the blood vessel) (see also 'myocardial infarction')

diuretic A drug which increases the volume of water lost from the body in the urine. Diuretics may be prescribed to treat any disorder of the heart, kidneys or liver which has resulted in excessive fluid retention

ECG (electrocardiogram) A recording of the electrical activity in the heart muscle associated with the contraction and relaxation of the atria and ventricles during each heartbeat. An ECG, which may be displayed on a monitor or traced out on a strip of paper, can be used to diagnose heart disease or to detect an abnormal heart rhythm

enzyme A protein which speeds up a chemical reaction without itself being altered by that reaction; the many thousands of enzymes in the human body are essential for the cells, tissues and organs to survive and function normally

epididymis The highly coiled tube (around seven metres long) at the back of each testicle which connects it to the vas deferens

expectorant An ingredient found in some cough remedies which makes it easier to cough up sputum, usually by causing the secretions inside the airways to become thinner and less sticky

faeces Waste material from the digestive tract which is normally eliminated from the body through the anus. Faeces consist of undigested food (mainly cellulose), bacteria (dead and alive), cells from the bowel lining, secretions from glands in the bowel lining, bile from the liver and water

fat The most highly concentrated source of energy from food, each gram of fat provides around 38 Calories, about twice as much energy as a gram of carbohydrate. There are three types of fat – saturated, polyunsaturated and mono-unsaturated – which vary in their chemical composition and effects on the body. Saturated fats are found in animal and dairy products; polyunsaturated fats are extracted from plant seeds, for example sunflower, safflower and soya bean; mono-unsaturated fats are found mainly in olives, peanuts and avocados. Too much of any type of fat increases the risk of obesity. However, saturated fat is also linked with heart disease because it increases the levels of cholesterol (see page 305) in the bloodstream

fibre The indigestible parts of plant foods, such as grain husks, the skin and flesh of fruits and the tough fibrous material in vegetables. Although fibre has no nutritional or energy value, it is an essential ingredient in a healthy diet because it helps prevent constipation, regulates the absorption of sugar and digested fats, and can slightly lower blood cholesterol

gastritis Inflammation of the stomach lining. Acute (see page 301) gastritis may cause abdominal discomfort, nausea and vomiting and can be due to excessive alcohol consumption, aspirin usage or a viral infection. Chronic (see page 305) gastritis, as a result of, for example, smoking or alcohol abuse, may not cause any symptoms and may only be discovered during an investigation for some other disorder

haemoglobin An iron-containing pigment (haem) combined with a protein (globin) which gives red blood cells their colour and enables them to pick up oxygen in the lungs and release oxygen as they pass through other parts of the body

haemophilia An inherited blood-clotting disorder caused by an abnormal gene, which results in a life-long tendency to bleed excessively following a minor injury or to bleed spontaneously, for example into joints or muscles. There are two types of haemophilia: the most common type, haemophilia A, is due to a lack of clotting factor VIII. Haemophilia B (often referred to as Christmas disease, taking its name from the surname of the first child to be identified with this condition) is due to lack of clotting factor IX. About 5,400 people in the UK have haemophilia A and about 1,100 have haemophilia B. Treatment involves regular injections of the missing clotting factor, obtained either from donated blood or as a synthetic product manufactured from DNA grown artificially in cell cultures

heart attack See 'coronary thrombosis' and 'myocardial infarction'

Helicobacter pylori (H. pylori) Spiral-shaped bacteria that can infect and damage the lining of the stomach and duodenum causing a peptic ulcer (see page 310), and possibly also cancer of the stomach. Management of a peptic ulcer nowadays will usually include a blood or breath test or a biopsy of the ulcer to see if H. pylori are present. To cure a peptic ulcer successfully in someone with this infection, a course of antibiotics will be prescribed in addition to an ulcer-healing drug.

hiatus hernia See 'acid reflux'

HIV-positive Possessing antibodies to Human Immunodeficiency Virus in the blood. People who are HIV-positive are often completely free of symptoms of ill health, but can pass on the infection to others, for example through unprotected sexual intercourse or sharing a needle

hyperglycaemia Abnormally high levels of sugar in the bloodstream, occurring in untreated diabetes or if a diabetic eats too many sugary foods and/or is not taking enough medication. Symptoms include drowsiness, acetone odour on the breath, confusion and, in severe cases, lapsing into a coma

hypertension Abnormally high blood pressure

hypoglycaemia Abnormally low levels of sugar in the bloodstream, most common in diabetics who have taken too high a dose of medication or too little carbohydrate food. Symptoms include nausea, dizziness, sweating, weakness, loss of co-ordination and confusion (see also 'reactive hypoglycaemia')

incontinence Uncontrolled, unwanted loss of urine, much rarer in men than in women. In men, urinary incontinence is usually caused by obstruction of the normal urine outflow by an enlarged prostate gland. Incontinence of faeces, where a man becomes unable to control his bowel movements, is generally confined to older men and may be caused by severe or long-standing constipation

insulin A hormone released into the bloodstream from the pancreas gland which stimulates the uptake of glucose (sugar) from the circulation into cells throughout the body and also influences the chemical processing of carbohydrates, fats and proteins. A deficiency or absence of insulin causes diabetes mellitus (see pages 218–20)

keratin A fibrous protein found in hair, nails and the outer layers of skin

lymph Fluid within the lymphatic system (see pages 46–7)

metabolism The various chemical and physical processes occurring inside the body which result in energy production from nutrients (catabolism) and the growth and repair of tissues and organs from molecular building blocks (anabolism)

minerals Chemical elements needed in the diet, usually only in small amounts, to maintain good health. Minerals known to play a key role in cell function include calcium, iron, potassium, sodium and zinc

mucus A sticky fluid, produced by glands in the membranes lining many different parts of the body, which has a protective and lubricating function

myocardial infarction A heart attack in which part of the heart muscle (myocardium) dies

neurosis A mental illness where there is abnormal behaviour or thinking, but where the individual remains in touch with reality and has some insight into his condition

nicotine An addictive ingredient in tobacco, which in small doses can have a slight stimulating effect on mood. Although not generally as harmful as some of the other toxic substances present within inhaled tobacco smoke, nicotine is likely to pose a health risk to people with high blood pressure or a circulation disorder because it causes narrowing of blood vessels

obesity Excess fat. In men, such fat is usually accumulated as an abdominal paunch. A person with a body mass index (BMI – weight in kg divided by the square of the height in metres) of over 30 is considered obese

osteoporosis Loss of bone substance causing the affected bones to become brittle and more vulnerable to fracture; it may be caused by poor diet, cigarette smoking, lack of exercise and high doses of steroids, and is much more common in women, particularly after the menopause, than in men

palpitation The sensation of becoming aware of your own heartbeat, most often in a situation where the heart has started to beat faster and more powerfully than normal (although it can also occur where there is no change in the heart rhythm or rate). Palpitations which last longer than a few minutes or which are recurrent can be a symptom of anxiety, a heart disorder or an over-active thyroid gland

peptic ulcer An erosion or crater in the lining of the duodenum, stomach or, more rarely, the oesophagus

peristalsis Spontaneous rhythmical contraction and relaxation of the muscles in the walls of various hollow tubes in the body to produce a wave-like movement

postnatal Occurring after birth

prostate gland A gland about the size of a chestnut, situated just below the bladder and in front of the rectum, which contributes nutrients and enzymes to the seminal fluid

protein An important nutrient, made up of thousands of chemical units known as amino acids (see page 302), which is obtained from animal and/or plant sources. Amino acids enable the body to make new proteins necessary for the growth, development, repair and maintenance of cells and tissues and the production of the various hormones and enzymes which regulate body function

psychosis Severe mental illness which may involve delusions, hallucinations, disturbed thought processes, grossly abnormal behaviour and/or extreme alterations in mood. Psychosis differs from neurosis in that the sufferer loses contact with reality and lacks insight into the seriousness of his condition

psychosomatic illness Any medical condition which may have been caused or made worse by psychological factors. It does not, as is often mistakenly thought, imply that the symptoms do not really exist, rather that an emotional factor, such as stress, may be a contributing factor

psychotherapy The use of psychological methods to treat an emotional, behavioural or mental disorder. There are various types of psychotherapy, all of which are based on the therapist establishing a relationship with the individual which encourages personal development and better self-awareness, thereby helping the patient resolve his conflicts and difficulties

radiotherapy The use of ionising radiation as a medical treatment, primarily used nowadays to shrink a cancerous tumour or reduce the chance of cancer spreading to other parts of the body

reactive hypoglycaemia A rapid fall in blood sugar due to a sudden release of large amounts of insulin by the pancreas gland responding to the digestion of sugar-rich food. It can be avoided by sticking to snacks that contain starches, fats or proteins rather than sugars (see also 'hypoglycaemia')

Reference Nutrient Intake (RNI) The quantity of a nutrient, such as vitamin C, which should be consumed each day to satisfy the nutritional needs of the average person (previously called the Recommended Daily Allowance)

saliva A slightly alkaline watery fluid released into the mouth by the three pairs of surrounding salivary glands, saliva is the body's natural antibacterial mouthwash, which also acts as a lubricant to assist chewing and swallowing and dissolves chemical particles in food, allowing them to be tasted

sebum An oily substance, released from the sebaceous glands within the skin, which helps keep the skin surface slightly moist and also has an antibacterial effect

semen Creamy, sticky fluid, produced mainly by the prostate gland and seminal vesicles, which is forcefully released from the urethral opening at the tip of the penis during ejaculation and which contains fructose and a variety of other nutrients to help keep sperm alive

septum Dividing wall between different areas of the body

sexually transmitted disease An infectious disease spread by sexual intercourse

sphincter A ring of muscle surrounding a passage or opening in the body, contraction of which will partly or completely close off that area

sputum Mucus produced by specialised cells within the lining of the bronchial airways which helps trap particles such as dust and smoke, thereby preventing them entering and damaging the lungs

suppository Medication in a solid form suitable for insertion into the rectum, where it slowly dissolves and releases its ingredients. Some suppositories have a local effect, for example to relieve constipation; others contain drugs which are absorbed into the general circulation to affect other parts of the body. They may be given to patients who have been vomiting to ensure the drug stays in the system

testosterone The most important of the male sex hormones (produced mainly by the testicles, but also in small amounts by the adrenal glands), testosterone stimulates muscle and bone development and is responsible for the secondary sexual characteristics which start to appear in young men at puberty (see pages 57–58)

tranquilliser A drug which produces a calming effect. Minor tranquillisers (such as the benzodiazepines) are used to treat anxiety and other neuroses; major tranquillisers (such as the phenothiazines) are used to treat schizophrenia and other psychoses

trans–urethral resection of the prostate (TURP) The commonest type of surgical operation for an enlarged prostate. A telescopic instrument is inserted into the urethra (under a general or spinal anaesthetic) and the obstruction cut away using an electrically heated wire loop

varicocele A varicose vein surrounding the testicle, usually the one on the left side of the scrotum

vas deferens A narrow tube that carries sperm from the epididymis at the back of the testicle to the urethra prior to ejaculation

vein A vessel carrying blood towards the heart. Veins have much thinner and less elastic walls than arteries (see page 303) because they are under much less pressure

vitamins Chemical compounds essential for health which cannot be made in the body, so must be obtained from the diet. The various roles of vitamins include stimulating the growth and repair of tissues, controlling chemical processes which release energy, and breaking down toxic substances which might otherwise cause cancer or heart disease

Addresses

Acne Support Group
PO Box 230, Hayes, Middlesex UB4 0UT
Email: alison@the_asg.demon.co.uk
Write enclosing sae

Action for M.E.
PO Box 1302, Wells, Somerset BA5 1YE
Tel: (01749) 670799
Fax: (01749) 672561
Web site: www.afme.org.uk

Action for Victims of Medical Accidents
Bank Chambers, 1 London Road,
London SE23 3TP
Tel: 0181-686 8333

Action on Smoking and Health (ASH)
16 Fitzhardinge Street, London W1H 9PL
Tel: 0171-224 0743
Fax: 0171-224 0471
Email: ash-uk@dial.pipex.com
Web site: www.ash.org.uk

AL-ANON
61 Great Dover Street, London SE1 4YF
Tel: 0171-403 0888
Fax: 0171-378 9910
Email: alanonuk@aol.com
Web site: www.hexnet.co.uk/alanon

Alcoholics Anonymous (AA)
General Service Office, PO Box 1,
Stonebow House, Stonebow, York,
North Yorkshire YO1 7NJ
Helpline: (0345) 697555 (*24 hours*)

Alzheimer's Disease Society
Gordon House, 10 Greencoat Place,
London SW1P 1PH
Tel: 0171-306 0606
Fax: 0171-306 0808
Email: info@alzheimers.org.uk
Web site: www.alzheimers.org.uk

Arthritis Care
18 Stephenson Way, London NW1 2HD
Tel: 0171-916 1500
Helpline: (0800) 289170 (*Mon–Fri,
12 noon–5pm*)
Fax: 0171-916 1505
Web site: www.vois.org.uk/arthritiscare

**Association for Spina Bifida and
Hydrocephalus (ASBAH)**
ASBAH House, 42 Park Road,
Peterborough, PE1 2UQ
Tel: (01733) 555988
Fax: (01733) 555985
Email: postmaster@asbah.demon.co.uk
Web site: www.asbah.demon.co.uk/

Birth Control Trust
16 Mortimer Street, London W1N 7RD
Tel: 0171-580 9360
Fax: 0171-637 1378
Email: bct@birthcontroltrust.org.uk
Web site: www.easynet.co.uk/bct

British Association of Cancer United Patients (BACUP)
3 Bath Place, Rivington Street,
London EC2A 3DR
Information service: (0800) 181199
Counselling service: 0171-696 9000
Fax: 0171-696 9002
Web site: www.cancerbacup.org.uk

British Association for Sexual and Marital Therapy
PO Box 13686, London SW20 9ZH
Email: BASMT@BASMT.demon.co.uk

British Cardiac Patients Association (Zipper Club)
c/o Keith Jackson, 6 Rampton End,
Willingham, Cambridge CB4 5JB
Tel/Fax: (01954) 202022
Helpline: (01223) 846845

British Chiropody Association
The SMAE Institute, The New Hall,
149 Bath Road, Maidenhead,
Berkshire SL6 4LA
Tel: (01628) 621100
Fax: (01628) 674483
Email:
SMAE_INSTITUTE@compuserve.com
Web site: ourworld.compuserve.com/
homepages/SMAE_INSTITUTE

British Colostomy Association
15 Station Road, Reading,
Berkshire RG1 1LG
Tel: 0118-9391537
Fax: 0118-956 9095
Helpline: (0800) 3284257
Email: sue@bcass.org.uk
Web site: www.bcass.org.uk

British Diabetic Association
10 Queen Anne Street,
London W1M 0BD
Careline: 0171-636 6112
Fax: 0171-637 3644
Email: bda@diabetes.org.uk
Web site: www.diabetes.org.uk/bda.htm

British Epilepsy Association
Anstey House, 40 Hanover Square,
Leeds LS3 1BE
Helpline: (0800) 309030
Fax: 0113-242 8804
Web site: www.epilepsy.org.uk/

British Heart Foundation
14 Fitzhardinge Street,
London W1H 4DH
Tel: 0171-935 0185
Information line: (0990) 200656
Fax: 0171-486 5820
Web site: www.bhf.org.uk

British Holistic Medical Association
Rowland Thomas House, Royal
Shrewsbury Hospital, South Shrewsbury,
Shropshire SY3 8XF
Tel/fax: (01273) 725951

British Red Cross Society
9 Grosvenor Crescent, London SW1X 7EJ
Tel: 0171-235 5454
Fax: 0171-245 6315
Email: information@redcross.org.uk
Web site: www.redcross.org.uk

British Wheel of Yoga
1 Hamilton Place, Boston Road, Sleaford,
Lincolnshire NG34 7ES
Fax: (01529) 303233
Email: wheelyoga@aol.com
Web site: members.aol.com/wheelyoga
Write enclosing an sae

Brook Advisory Centre
165 Gray's Inn Road,
London WC1X 8UD
Tel: 0171-833 8488
Fax: 0171-833 8182
Email: brookcentres@compuserve.com

CHILD
Charter House, 43 St Leonards Road,
Bexhill-on-Sea, East Sussex TN40 1JA
Tel: (01424) 732361
Fax: (01424) 731858
Email: office@email2.child.org.uk
Web site: www.child.org.uk

The Coeliac Society
PO Box 220, High Wycombe,
Buckinghamshire HP11 2HY
Tel: (01494) 437278
Fax: (01494) 474349
Email: admin@coeliac.co.uk
Web site: www.coeliac.co.uk

Contraception Education Service
2–12 Pentonville Road, London N1 9FP
Tel: 0171-837 4044
Fax: 0171-837 3034

The Coronary Prevention Group
42 Store Street, London WC1E 7DB
Tel: 0171-580 1070
Fax: 0171-436 6220
Web site: www.healthnet.org.uk

CRY-SIS
BM CRY-SIS, London WC1N 3XX
Tel: 0171-404 5011 (*24 hours*)

Depression Alliance
35 Westminster Bridge Road,
London SE1 7JB
Tel: 0171-633 9929 (*answerphone*)
Fax: 0171-633 0559
Web site: www.gn.apc.org/da/

Depressives Anonymous
36 Chestnut Avenue, Beverley,
East Yorkshire HU17 9QU
Tel: (01482) 860619
Fax: (01482) 887634
Web site: www.ribblewebdesign.co.uk/fda

Diabetes Foundation
177A Tennison Road, London SE25 5NF
Tel: 0181-656 5467 (*answerphone*)

Digestive Disorders Foundation
PO Box 251, Edgeware,
Middlesex HA8 6HG
Tel: 0171-487 5332 (*answerphone*)
Web site: www.digestivedisorders.org.uk

English Sports Council
16 Upper Woburn Place,
London WC1H 0QP
Tel: 0171-273 1500
Web site: www.english.sports.gov.uk
Provides a list of sports facilities in your area

Families Need Fathers
National Administration Centre,
134 Curtain Road, London EC2A 3AR
Tel: (0990) 502506 (*answerphone*)
Fax: 0171-739 3410
Web site: www.vix.com/fnf

Family Heart Association
7 North Road, Maidenhead,
Berkshire SL6 1PL
Tel: (01628) 628638
Fax: (01628) 628698
Email: family@heart.k-web.co.uk

Family Planning Association
2–12 Pentonville Road, London N1 9FP
Tel: 0171-837 5432
Helpline: 0171-837 4044
Fax: 0171-837 6785

Federation of Holistic Therapists
3rd Floor, Eastleigh House, Upper Market
Street, Eastleigh, Hampshire SO50 9FD
Tel: (01703) 488900
Fax: (01703) 488970
Email: gr34@dial.pipex.com

Fertility UK
Clitherow House, 1 Blythe Mews,
Blythe Road, London W14 0NW
Tel: 0171-371 1341
Fax: 0171-371 4921
Email: jknight@enterprise.net
Web site: www.FertilityUK.org/index.html

General Medical Council
178 Great Portland Street,
London W1N 6NH
Tel: 0171-580 7642
Fax: 0171-915 3641

Haemophilia Society
Chesterfield House, 385 Euston Road,
London NW1 3AU
Tel: 0171-380 0600
Fax: 0171-387 8220
Email: info@haemophilia-soc.demon.co.uk
Web site: www.haemophilia.org.uk

**Hairline International / The Alopecia
Patients' Society**
Lyons Court, 1668 High Street, Knowle,
Solihull, West Midlands B93 0LY
Tel: (01564) 775281 (*answerphone*)

**Headway (National Head Injuries
Association)**
4 King Edward Court, King Edward
Street, Nottingham NG1 1EW
Tel: 0115-9240800
Fax: 0115-9584446
Email: general@headway.org.uk
Web site: www.headway.org.uk

Health Advice for Travellers
Helpline: (0800) 555777

Health Education Authority
Trevelyan House, 30 Great Peter Street,
London SW1P 2BY
Tel: 0171-222 5300
Fax: 0171-413 8900
Web site: www.hea.org.uk

**Hearing Concern
(British Association of the Hard of
Hearing)**
7–11 Armstrong Road, London W3 7JL
Tel: 0181-743 1110
Helpline: (01245) 344600
Fax: 0181-742 9043
Email: hearing.concern@ukonline.co.uk
Web site: web.ukonline.co.uk/
hearing.concern/

Herpes Viruses Association
41 North Road, London N7 9DP
Helpline: 0171-609 9061

Human BSE Foundation Helpline
Tel: (01380) 720033

**Human Fertilisation and Embryology
Authority**
Paxton House, 30 Artillery Lane,
London E1 7LS
Tel: 0171-377 5077
Fax: 0171-377 1871
Web site: www.hfea.gov.uk

Impotence Association
PO Box 10296, London SW17 9WH
Tel: 0181-767 7791
Fax: 0181-516 7725

International Glaucoma Association
Kings College Hospital, Denmark Hill,
London SE5 9RS
Tel: 0171-737 3265
Fax: 0171-346 5929
Email: ita@kcl.ac.uk
Web site: www.ita.org.uk/iga/

ISSUE (National Fertility Association)
114 Lichfield Street, Walsall,
West Midlands WS1 1SZ
Tel: (01922) 722888
Fax: (01922) 640070
Email: webmaster@issue.co.uk
Web site: www.issue.co.uk

Macmillan Cancer Relief
Anchor House, 15–19 Britten Street,
London SW3 3TZ
Tel: 0171-351 7811
Information line: (0845) 6016161
(*9.30am–7.30pm*)
Fax: 0171-376 8098
Web site: www.macmillan.org.uk

Manic Depression Fellowship
8–10 High Street, Kingston-upon-Thames,
Surrey KT1 1EY
Tel: 0181-974 6550
Fax: 0181-974 6600

Men's Health Matters
Blythe Hall, 100 Blythe Road,
London W14 0HB
Advice line: 0181-995 4448 (*6pm–10pm*)

Migraine Action Association
178 High Road, Byfleet, West Byfleet,
Surrey KT14 7ED
Tel: (01932) 352468
Fax: (01932) 351257
Email: info@migraine.org.uk
Web site: www.migraine.org.uk

Migraine Trust
45 Great Ormond Street,
London WC1N 3HZ
Tel: 0171-831 4818
Fax: 0171-831 5174

**MIND (National Association for
Mental Health)**
Granta House, 15–19 Broadway, Stratford,
London E15 4BQ
Tel: 0181-519 2122 (ext. 275)
Helpline: (0345) 660163 *(for callers outside
London; calls are charged at local rates)*
Fax: 0181-522 1725
Email: contact@mind.org.uk
Web site: www.mind.org.uk

Multiple Sclerosis Society
25 Effie Road, London SW6 1EE
Tel: 0171-736 6267
Fax: 0171-736 7861
Email: info@mssociety.org.uk
Web site: www.mssociety.org.uk

Myalgic Encephalomyelitis Association
4 Corringham Road, Stanford-le-Hope,
Essex SS17 0AH
Tel: (01375) 642466 *(10am–4pm)*
Information line: (01375) 361013
(1.30pm–4pm)
Fax: (01375) 360256

National AIDS Helpline
Tel: (0800) 567123 *(24 hours)*

**National Association for Colitis and
Crohn's Disease**
4 Beaumont House, Sutton Road,
St Albans, Hertfordshire AL1 5HH
Tel: (01727) 844296
Fax: (01727) 862550
Email: nacc@nacc.org.uk
Web site: www.nacc.org.uk

National Association of Deafened People
c/o Jenny Dunning, Ashby Place,
26 Stubbs Wood, Chesham Bois,
Buckinghamshire HP6 6EY
Tel: (0494) 724830

National Asthma Campaign
Providence House, Providence Place,
London N1 0NT
Tel: 0171-226 2260
Fax: 0171-704 0740
Helpline: (0345) 010203 *(daily, 9am–7pm)*
Web site: www.asthma.org.uk

National Back Pain Association
16 Elmtree Road, Teddington,
Middlesex TW11 8FT
Email: 101540.1065@compuserve.com
Web site: www.backpain.org/
Information pack available for £2.50 p&p

National CJD Support Network
Tel/fax: (01630) 673973

National Eczema Society
163 Eversholt Street, London NW1 1BU
Tel: 0171-388 4097
Helpline: 0171-388 4800
Fax: 0171-388 5882
Web site: www.eczema.org

National Osteoporosis Society
PO Box 10, Radstock, Bath BA3 3YB
Tel: (01761) 471771
Helpline: (01761) 472721
Fax: (01761) 471104
Email: info@nos.org.uk
Web site: www.nos.org.uk

National Sports Medicine Institute
Charterhouse Square, London EC1M 6BQ
Tel: 0171-251 0583
Fax: 0171-251 0774
Email: nsmi@mds.qmw.ac.uk
Web site: www.nsmi.org.uk/

NORM UK
PO Box 71, Stone, Staffordshire ST15 0SF
Tel/fax: (01785) 814044 *(answerphone)*

The Parkinson's Disease Society
215 Vauxhall Bridge Road,
London SW1V 1EJ
Tel: 0171-931 8080
Helpline: 0171-233 5373
Fax: 0171-233 9908

Prostate Cancer Charity
Du Cane Road, London W12 0NN
Helpline: 0181-383 1948
Fax: 0181-383 8126
Email: n.roberts@rpms.ac.uk
Web site: www.prostate-cancer.org.uk/

Prostate Help Association
Langworth, Lincoln LN3 5DF
Send two first class stamps for information

Prostate Research Campaign
36 The Drive, Northwood, Middlesex
HA6 1HP
Send large sae for information

Psoriasis Association
7 Milton Street, Northampton,
Northamptonshire NN2 7JG
Tel: (01604) 711129
Fax: (01604) 792894

Quitline
Tel: (0800) 002200
Counsellors offer advice to anyone trying to stop smoking; daily, 9am–11pm

Relate
Herbert Gray College, Little Church
Street, Rugby, Warwicks CV21 3AP
Tel: (01788) 573241
Fax: (01788) 535007
Email: info@relate.org.uk
Web site: www.relate.org.uk

Release
388 Old Street, London EC1V 9LT
Advice line: 0171-729 9904 (*10am–6pm*)
Advice line: 0171-603 8654 (*after hours*)
Fax: 0171-729 2599
Email: info@release.org.uk
Web site: www.release.org.uk

Royal National Institute for the Blind (RNIB)
224 Great Portland Street,
London W1N 6AA
Tel: 0171-388 1266
Helpline: (0345) 669999
(*Mon–Fri, 9am–5pm*)
Fax: 0171-388 2034
Email: Helpline@rnib.org.uk
Web site: www.rnib.org.uk/

Royal National Institute for Deaf People (RNID)
19–23 Featherstone Street,
London EC1Y 8SL
Tel: (0870) 6050123 (*9.30am–5pm*)
Textline: (0870) 6033007 (*9.30am–5pm*)
Fax: 0171-296 8199
Email: helpline@RNID.org.uk
Web site: www.rnid.org.uk
Write to PO Box 16464, London
EC1Y 8TT for information

RSI Association
Chapel House, 152 High Street, Yiewsley,
West Drayton, Middlesex UB7 7BE
Tel: (01895) 431134 (*Mon–Fri, 2pm–4pm*)
Fax: (01895) 437300

SAD (Seasonal Affective Disorder) Association
PO Box 989, Steyning,
West Sussex BN44 3HG
Tel: (01903) 814942
Fax: (01903) 879939

Samaritans
General Office, 10 The Grove, Slough,
Berkshire SL1 1QP
Tel: (01753) 216500
Helpline: (0345) 909090 (*24 hours*)
Fax: (01753) 819004
Email: jo@samaritans.org.uk (*enables you to send an anonymous email*)
Web site: www.samaritans.org.uk/

Society of Chiropodists
53 Wellbeck Street, London W1M 7HE
Tel: 0171-486 3381
Fax: 0171-835 6359

Spinal Injuries Association
76 St James's Lane, London N10 3DF
Tel: 0181-444 2121
Counselling line: 0181-883 4296
(*Mon–Fri, 2–5pm*)
Fax: 0181-444 3761
Email: sia@spinali.demon.co.uk
Web site: jgrweb.com/sia/

Standing Conference on Drug Abuse (SCODA)
Waterbridge House, 32–36 Loman Street,
London SE1 0EE
Tel: 0171-928 9500
Fax: 0171-928 3343
Email: info@scoda.demon.co.uk
Web site: www.ncvo-vol.org.uk/scoda.html

St John Ambulance
1 Grosvenor Crescent, London SW1X 7EF
Tel: 0171-235 5231
Fax: 0171-235 0796

Stroke Association
Stroke House, 123–127 Whitecross Street,
London EC1Y 8JJ
Tel: 0171-566 0300
Fax: 0171-490 2686
Email: stroke@stroke.org.uk
Website: www.stroke.org.uk

Tenovus Cancer Information Centre
College Building, Courtenay Road, Splott,
Cardiff CF1 1SA
Tel: (01222) 497700
Fax: (01222) 489919
Helpline: (0800) 526527 (*Mon–Fri,
9–4.30pm; answerphone at other times*)
Email: tcicancer@aol.com

Terrence Higgins Trust
52–54 Gray's Inn Road,
London WC1X 8JU
Tel: 0171-831 0330
Fax: 0171-242 0121
Helpline: 0171-242 1010
(*daily, 12 noon–10pm*)
Legal line: 0171-405 2381
(*Mon and Wed, 7–9pm*)
Email: info@tht.org.uk
Web site: www.tht.org.uk

Transcendental Meditation (TM)
Beacon House, Willow Walk,
Skelmersdale, Lancashire WN8 6SW
Tel: (0990) 143733
Fax: (01695) 727499
Email: tminfo@maharishi.org.uk
Web site: www.transcendental-meditation.org.uk

Uncircumcising Information Resources Centre (UNCIRC)
PO Box 52138, Pacific Grove, California
93950, USA
Tel/Fax: +1 408 375 4326

Yoga for Health Foundation
Ickwell Bury, Biggleswade,
Bedfordshire SG18 9EF
Tel: (01767) 627271
Fax: (01767) 627266

Publications

How to cope with sleep problems leaflet
Mind Publications, 15–19 Broadway,
Stratford, London E15 4BQ
Send £1 postal order, plus 38p A5 sae

Insomnia information pack
Sleep Matters, PO Box 3087,
London W4 4ZP
Send £3 postal order

Bibliography

The following is a short list of books which offer further information on various topics covered within the text.

Zilbergeld, Dr B. 1980 *Men and Sex – A Guide to Sexual Fulfilment* (Fontana)

Masters, Dr W. & Johnson Dr V. 1966 *Human Sexual Response* (Little, Brown, out of print)

Lacroix, N. 1989 *Sensual Massage – An Intimate and Practical Guide to the Art of Touch* (Dorling Kindersley)

Isay, R. A. 1993 *Being Homosexual – Gay Men and Their Development* (Penguin)

Weeks, J. 1991 *Against Nature – Essays on History, Sexuality and Identity (Rivers Oram Press)*

Llewellyn-Jones, Dr D. 1991 *Everyman* (Oxford University Press)

Smith, Dr T. 1990 *British Medical Association Complete Family Health Encyclopaedia* (Dorling Kindersley)

Youngson, Dr R. M. 1992 *Collins Dictionary of Medicine* (HarperCollins)

Carroll Dr S. 1992 *The Complete Family Guide to Healthy Living* (Dorling Kindersley)

LaFavore, M. 1992 *Men's Health Advisor* (Rodale Press Inc.)

Pesman, P./*Esquire* Editors 1984 *How a Man Ages – Growing Older: What to Expect and What You Can Do About It* (Esquire Press)

Combes, G. & Schonveld, A. 1992 *Life Will Never Be The Same Again: Learning to be a First Time Parent* (Health Education Authority)

Braun, D. & Schonveld, A. 1993 *Approaching Parenthood Resource for Parent Education* (Health Education Authority)

Health Education Authority 1993 *A Complete Guide to Pregnancy, Childbirth and the First Few Weeks With a New Baby* (Health Education Authority)

Voluntary Agencies Directory 1993/4 (NVCO Publications, incorporating Bedford Square Press, 1993)

Wellings, K. et al 1993 *Sexual Behaviour in Britain* (Penguin)

Index